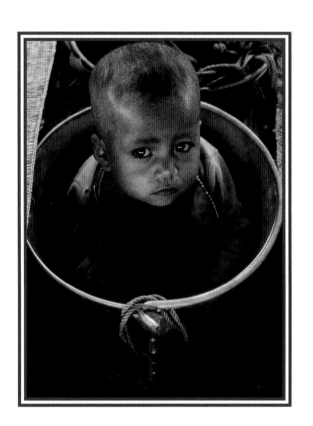

"my heart it
is delicious"

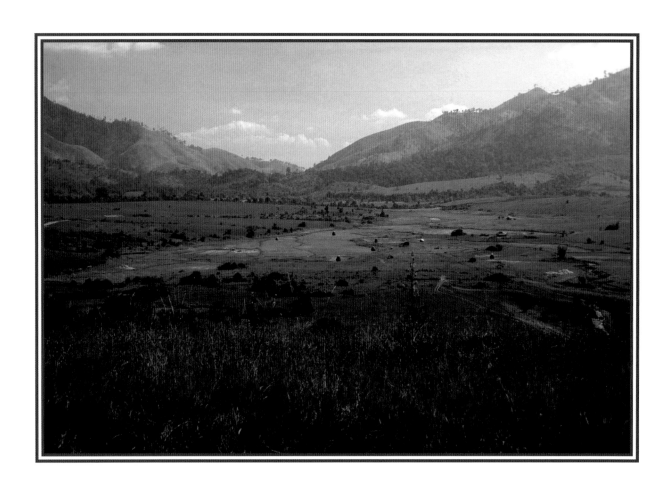

"my heart it is delicious"

setting the course for
cross-cultural health care

the story of the
CENTER FOR
INTERNATIONAL
HEALTH

biloine w. young
foreword by david etzwiler

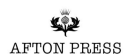

AFTON PRESS

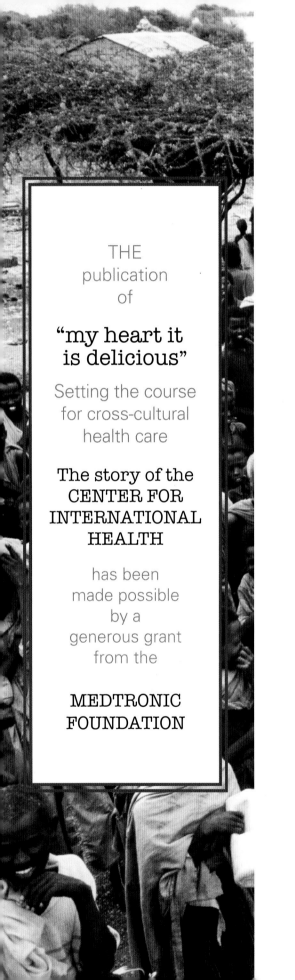

THE
publication
of

"my heart it is delicious"

Setting the course
for cross-cultural
health care

The story of the CENTER FOR INTERNATIONAL HEALTH

has been
made possible
by a
generous grant
from the

MEDTRONIC FOUNDATION

FRONT COVER: A young Ghanaian girl wears her finest clothes as she waits to see American doctors.

OPPOSITE HALF-TITLE PAGE: Parents carried their year-old baby in a bucket across the fields of Cambodia to safety in Thailand. Because of the long confinement, the child could not stand on arrival at the refugee camp hospital.

FRONTISPIECE: Phonsavan, Laos: view of mountains looking toward the Ho Chi Minh Trail.

PAGE 8: Dr. Pat Walker plays guitar in the company of Cambodian refugee Yong Yuth Banrith outside the American Refugee Committee (ARC) Ward 1 hospital in Khao I Dang camp, Thailand.

Edited by Michele Hodgson
Designed by Mary Susan Oleson
Production assistance by Beth Williams
Printed by Pettit Network Inc., Afton, Minnesota

Library of Congress Cataloging-in-Publication Data

Young, Biloine W., 1926-
  My heart it is delicious : setting the course for cross-cultural health care : the story of the Center for International Health / by Biloine Whiting Young.—1st ed.
    p. ; cm.
  ISBN-13: 978-1-890434-76-2 (hardcover : alk. paper)
  ISBN-10: 1-890434-76-0 (hardcover : alk. paper)
1. Center for International Health (Saint Paul, Minn.)—History. 2. American Refugee Committee (Minneapolis, Minn.)—History. 3. Transcultural medical care--Minnesota—History. 4. Refugees--Medical care—Minnesota—History. 5. Immigrants—Medical care—Minnesota—History. 6. Southeast Asians—Medical care—Minnesota—History. I. Title. [DNLM: 1. Center for International Health (Saint Paul, Minn.) 2.American Refugee Committee (Minneapolis, Minn.) 3. Delivery of Health Care—Asia, Southeastern. 4. Delivery of Health Care—Minnesota. 5.Refugees—psychology—Asia, Southeastern. 6. Refugees—psychology—Minnesota. 7. Cross-Cultural Comparison—Asia, Southeastern. 8. Cross-Cultural Comparison—Minnesota. 9. Emigration and Immigration—Asia, Southeastern. 10. Emigration and Immigration--Minnesota. 11. Health Services Accessibility—Asia, Southeastern. 12. Health Services Accessibility—Minnesota. WA 300 Y68m 2007]

 RA418.5.T73Y68 2007
 362.109776--dc22

                         2007026733
Printed in China

Afton Press receives major support for its publishing program from the Sarah Stevens MacMillan Foundation and the W. Duncan MacMillan family.

Patricia Condon McDonald
Publisher

AFTON HISTORICAL SOCIETY PRESS
P.O. Box 100, Afton, MN 55001   800-436-8443
aftonpress@aftonpress.com
www.aftonpress.com

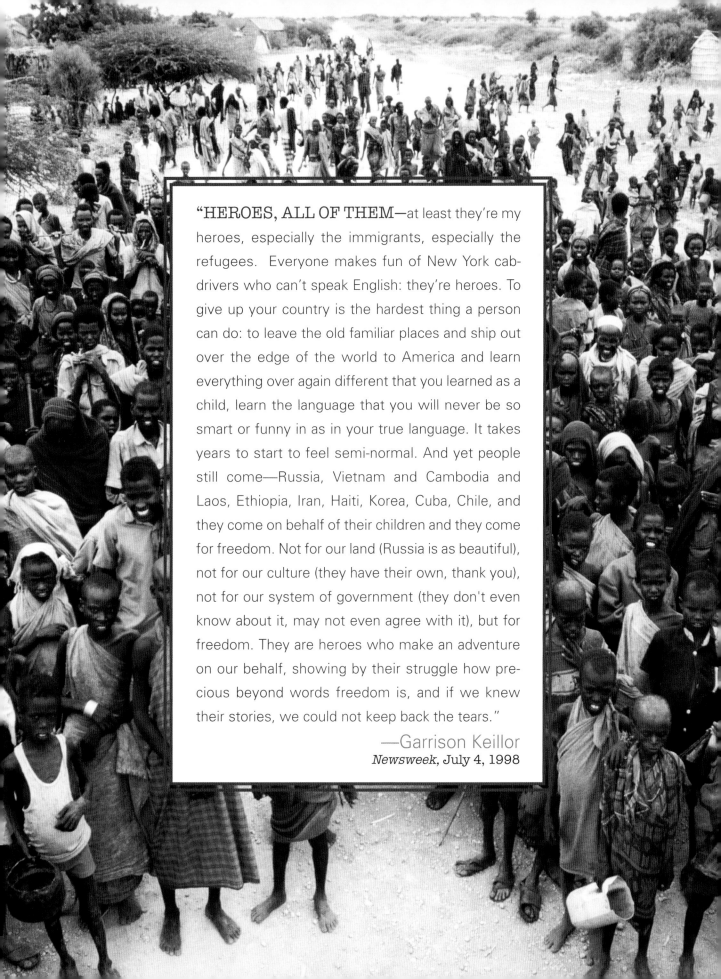

"HEROES, ALL OF THEM—at least they're my heroes, especially the immigrants, especially the refugees. Everyone makes fun of New York cab-drivers who can't speak English: they're heroes. To give up your country is the hardest thing a person can do: to leave the old familiar places and ship out over the edge of the world to America and learn everything over again different that you learned as a child, learn the language that you will never be so smart or funny in as in your true language. It takes years to start to feel semi-normal. And yet people still come—Russia, Vietnam and Cambodia and Laos, Ethiopia, Iran, Haiti, Korea, Cuba, Chile, and they come on behalf of their children and they come for freedom. Not for our land (Russia is as beautiful), not for our culture (they have their own, thank you), not for our system of government (they don't even know about it, may not even agree with it), but for freedom. They are heroes who make an adventure on our behalf, showing by their struggle how pre-cious beyond words freedom is, and if we knew their stories, we could not keep back the tears."

—Garrison Keillor
Newsweek, July 4, 1998

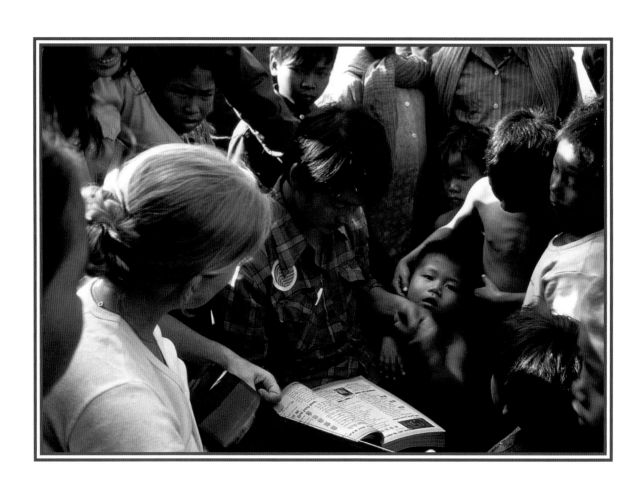

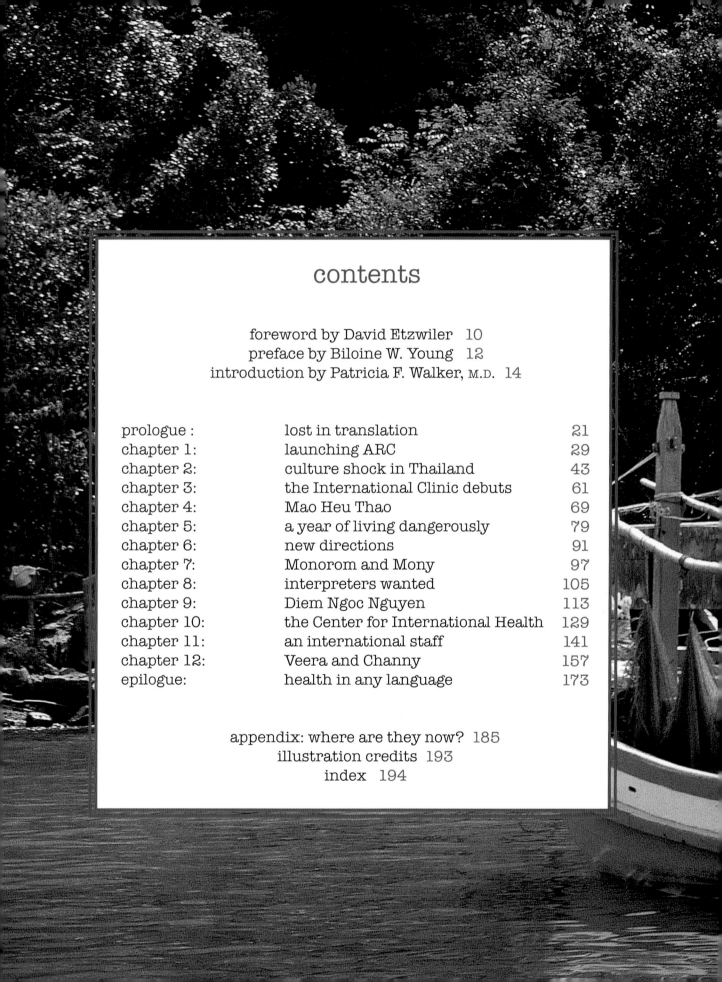

contents

foreword

I LOVE MY JOB.

That personal declaration may be an unorthodox opening to a book addressing cultural competency in health care, yet it neatly sums up the privilege I have in meeting many of the world's most interesting, intelligent, and compassionate people. People who are dedicated to making the world better, driven to "do the right thing." People like Dr. Pat Walker, who has changed the way we think about medicine.

It's often easy to think of health-care issues by the numbers—scientific studies and demographic statistics that identify problems and progress. All of this is absolutely critical in a never-ending quest to improve people's lives by ensuring they receive the best health care. But medicine is a one-on-one experience, and our challenge is to always put the person above collective patient data.

From her first days as part of a small but earnest medical team serving Cambodian refugee camps in the late 1970s, Dr. Walker has known the person behind the patient. Her firsthand experiences in Southeast Asia, coupled with new waves of immigrants and refugees looking for a haven in the United States and landing in strange places like Minnesota, set in motion a series of events that helped launch St. Paul's Center for International Health. A new medical discipline, focused on culturally competent care, was born.

In chronicling the development of the Center for International Health, now a nationally recognized model of immigrant care, *My Heart It Is Delicious* captures the stories of people seeking care in a foreign land. Through these stories, we find that the immigrants' cultural perspective on health care led to clashes with recommendations of traditionally trained U.S. physicians.

Be assured, this book criticizes neither doctors nor the immigrant patients they treat. Medical care is a two-way street, with both patient and doctor bringing responsibilities, background, and biases to the examining room. These stories, however, vividly demonstrate how language, income, family, and unfamiliarity with U.S. health systems can create a deep and treacherous cultural chasm. These are timeless stories that need to be told, helping us to understand and appreciate perspectives we may never have considered. These also are personal stories that introduce us to new neighbors, reward us with a deeper understanding of our global community, and teach us how to better care for each other.

The good news is that we are helping more people than ever before. The best practices, ideas, and philosophies developed at the Center for International Health—for example, something as basic and essential as translating drug prescription instructions—*have* changed the way we think and, more important, the way we care for people of varied cultural backgrounds. But the chasm still exists. I hope this book can bring this knowledge to an even greater audience of physicians, nurses, administrators, and patients—to anyone involved in our health-care system.

I'm proud that the Medtronic Foundation supports these efforts, which directly help advance our mission to bring equal health-care access to people who historically have been underserved. And I love my job because, in a small way, we help fuel the compassionate fire in people like Dr. Walker, which in turn improves health care one person at time.

David Etzwiler
EXECUTIVE DIRECTOR
Medtronic Foundation

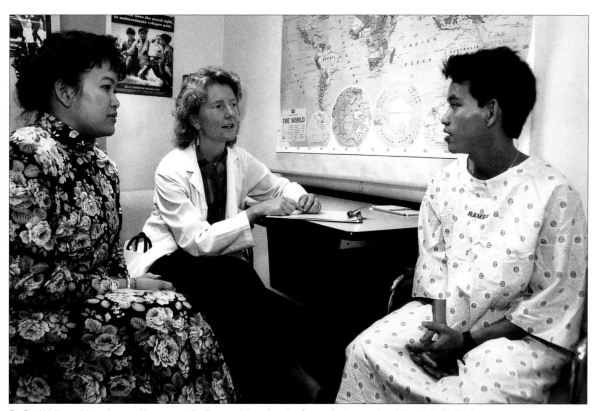

Dr. Pat Walker with patient and interpreter (in flowered dress) at the Center for International Health in St. Paul.

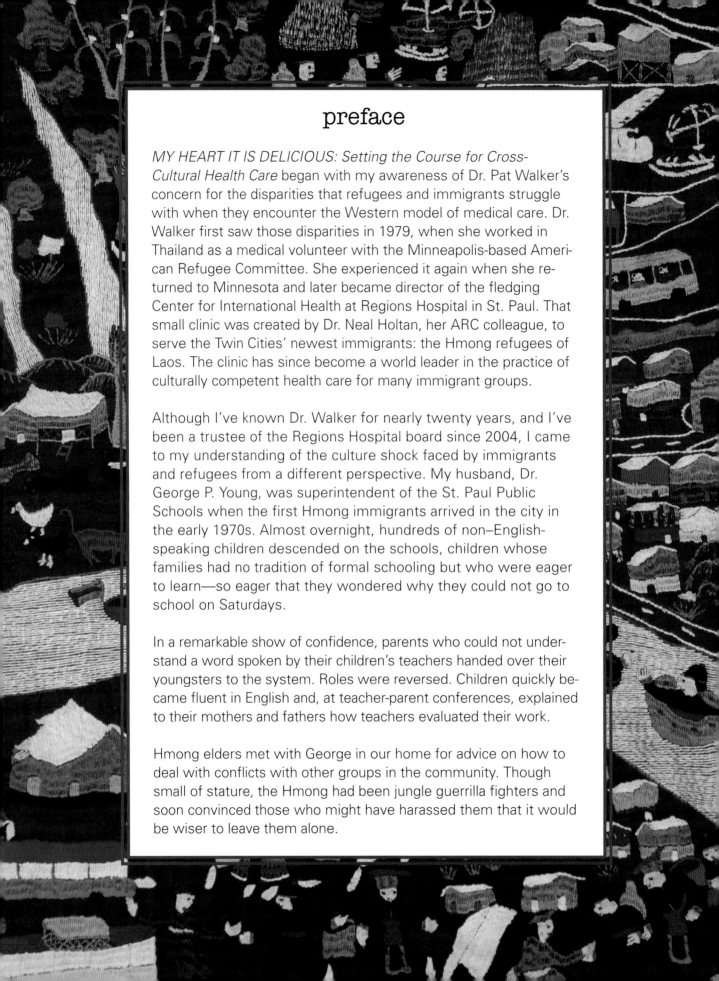

preface

MY HEART IT IS DELICIOUS: Setting the Course for Cross-Cultural Health Care began with my awareness of Dr. Pat Walker's concern for the disparities that refugees and immigrants struggle with when they encounter the Western model of medical care. Dr. Walker first saw those disparities in 1979, when she worked in Thailand as a medical volunteer with the Minneapolis-based American Refugee Committee. She experienced it again when she returned to Minnesota and later became director of the fledging Center for International Health at Regions Hospital in St. Paul. That small clinic was created by Dr. Neal Holtan, her ARC colleague, to serve the Twin Cities' newest immigrants: the Hmong refugees of Laos. The clinic has since become a world leader in the practice of culturally competent health care for many immigrant groups.

Although I've known Dr. Walker for nearly twenty years, and I've been a trustee of the Regions Hospital board since 2004, I came to my understanding of the culture shock faced by immigrants and refugees from a different perspective. My husband, Dr. George P. Young, was superintendent of the St. Paul Public Schools when the first Hmong immigrants arrived in the city in the early 1970s. Almost overnight, hundreds of non–English-speaking children descended on the schools, children whose families had no tradition of formal schooling but who were eager to learn—so eager that they wondered why they could not go to school on Saturdays.

In a remarkable show of confidence, parents who could not understand a word spoken by their children's teachers handed over their youngsters to the system. Roles were reversed. Children quickly became fluent in English and, at teacher-parent conferences, explained to their mothers and fathers how teachers evaluated their work.

Hmong elders met with George in our home for advice on how to deal with conflicts with other groups in the community. Though small of stature, the Hmong had been jungle guerrilla fighters and soon convinced those who might have harassed them that it would be wiser to leave them alone.

The Hmong, who were the first wave of latter-day ethnic groups to migrate to the United States and the Twin Cities, have since been joined by Vietnamese, Cambodian, Somali, Russian, Haitian, and Central American immigrants. As a result of Dr. Walker's efforts, doctors and nurses at the Center for International Health now look and speak more like the people they treat. Interpreters help bridge the gap between an immigrant's understanding of illness and a Western physician's methods of healing.

Chance and fate dictated that a group of well-intentioned Minnesotans, responding to a crisis half a world away, would be the spark that would ignite this new concept in health care, a way to practice medicine that is genuinely cross-cultural. This book is the story of the remarkable people who brought that concept about.

It was only through the willingness and generosity of the victims of the last century's violent upheavals that I was able to tell the story of the Center for International Health and its worldwide impact on the health care of refugees and immigrants. For sharing their past experiences I am grateful to Diem Ngoc Nguyen, who spent more than a month of Sundays over coffee in his dining room with me, his fingers nervously folding and refolding his napkin as he recalled devastating incidents from twelve years of imprisonment in North Vietnam. Sisters Veera and Channy Som also relived for my tape recorder their years as survivors of the murderous Pol Pot regime in Cambodia and as illegal residents of a refugee camp in Thailand. For their gift of time I am also grateful to Karen Johnson Elshazly of the American

Refugee Committee; Drs. Neal Holtan, Steve Miles, Kathleen Culhane-Pera, Mikhail Perelman, Fozia Abrar, Karen Ta, and Bruce Field; and Neal Ball, Bridget Votel, Glenda Potter, Monica Overkamp, Susan Walker, Elizabeth Walker Anderson, Barbara Huwe, Yong Yuth Banrith, Monorom Sok Hang, Mao Heu Thao, and May Mua.

I am deeply indebted to Dr. Pat Walker, medical director of St. Paul's Center for International Health, whose decision to interrupt her studies as a third-year medical student to work in a refugee camp in Thailand not only determined the trajectory of her own career, but influenced the way medical treatment would be provided for refugees and immigrants throughout the Western world. My thanks go as well to her entire staff, who put up with my days of leaning against a wall of the clinic corridor, notebook in hand, observing their activity. Conni Conner, senior administrative assistant at the Center for International Health, who was my covert ally in this project, has my profound gratitude for her ability to provide needed information, as well as to calm my Type A propensities when they threatened to get out of hand.

I am also most grateful to Chuck Johnston and Patricia McDonald of Afton Historical Society Press, who immediately grasped the message of this book and arranged for its publication; to Mary Sue Oleson, whose design illuminates the story in ways that words cannot; and to Michele Hodgson, whose editing makes every writer look good.

Biloine W. Young
ST. PAUL, MINNESOTA
March 2007

introduction

MRINAL PATNAIK was a confident young physician, at the top of his graduating class at Grant Medical College in Mumbai, India. Having won seven gold medals for his academic achievements, he was universally recognized by his peers for his brilliance. By his own admission, Mrinal was focused more on his career successes and less on the life stories of his patients. "I must admit I had developed a certain arrogance about me," he says.

After graduation, Mrinal was assigned to a compulsory two-month term of service in a village near Mumbai. The change in culture was dramatic. "I came from the big city," he recalls. "I was so shocked by the poverty."

One day, while listening to a young girl's chest, Mrinal heard a rumbling murmur that indicated mitral stenosis, an eventually fatal heart valve blockage. Mitral stenosis is often found in residents of poor rural areas of the world that lack access to simple penicillins. More than likely the girl had had strep throat as a child; left untreated, it had caused rheumatic fever, which infected her heart and kidneys.

"You must take your daughter to Mumbai to have open heart surgery to replace her mitral valve," Mrinal told the girl's mother. She had never gone to the next village, much less to the big city. "The next day she told me, 'I have sold my house and land, my jewelry, and my bullocks. I am ready to go to Mumbai for my daughter's surgery. How do I do this?"

"How much money do you have?" Mrinal asked, knowing the surgery would cost 80,000 rupees.

"One thousand rupees," she replied.

Mrinal was filled with remorse. "My advice had caused this mother to sell all her worldly belongings. I had changed their lives completely with my quick words the previous day." Deeply affected by the experience, Mrinal went back to Mumbai when his two-month stint was finished with his mind made up: instead of going to

America for his residency training, he would first spend a year as a village doctor. His middle-class parents, who had nurtured his education as well as that of his brothers, were disappointed, but Mrinal stuck with his plan. He was assigned to Raigod, a village in Maharashetra state, as a medical and snake bite officer for a vast rural area of forty thousand people. He was the sole physician, with a tiny staff of one pharmacist, four nurses, a malaria medical officer, and a leprosy medical officer.

"I actually almost didn't last the first day," Mrinal says, remembering the first time he had to fetch water from a stream and pump it through a handheld filter. "But I had to prove to my father that I could do it."

Since kerosene lanterns were the only light source after dark, most people went to bed with the sun. "At night, truth be told, I was actually bored," he says. "So I decided to go out into the hills to visit patients in their huts." One night he was awakened to tend to a patient and was upset that they would bother to disturb him. As he walked down the path lit only with lanterns, he heard the tinkle of cow bells and saw a woman in obstructed labor who had traveled on a bullock cart for twelve hours to see him, her husband walking alongside. "I felt so humbled by her terrible suffering, and shamed by my feelings. To have such experiences daily for a year was a turning point in my life."

Mrinal learned what life was really like for his patients: poverty so pervasive that parents were forced to choose between medications for illnesses and food or education for the children. The young physician decided to not charge his patients. Soon word

got around: "The doctor comes to see you in your home! He accepts no payments!"

He made sure that patients with tuberculosis and leprosy were getting their medications. He looked vigilantly for cases of measles and acute flaccid paralysis, a sign of a possible polio outbreak. Through his involvement with the World Health Organization, he treated people afflicted with guinea worm, which grows up to three feet and erupts through the skin, causing intense pain. Afflicted farmers cannot work in the fields; parents cannot care for their children; children miss school. The only treatment is to remove the worm over many weeks by winding it around a stick and pulling it out slowly. Keeping the larvae out of drinking water is the key to eliminating the worm.

Mrinal soon learned that health is not the first concern of the poor: water, food, safety, and shelter take precedence. He pitched in with various agriculture projects, helping to design small dams and irrigation ditches to improve crop yields, knowing that better nutrition meant better health. "I can tell you where I learned to care," he says. "It wasn't in medical school. It wasn't in my internal medicine residency at the University of Minnesota. It was my year in the village in India."

Mrinal told me this story one day while we sat in the Center for International Health. Like Mrinal, I had learned firsthand the reality of health care for many migrants. When I was a volunteer in Cambodian refugee camps, I saw the pervasive relationship of public health to poverty, religion, and politics, and the enormity of the tragedy that often befalls innocent people caught in the middle. I first met Mrinal when he asked to

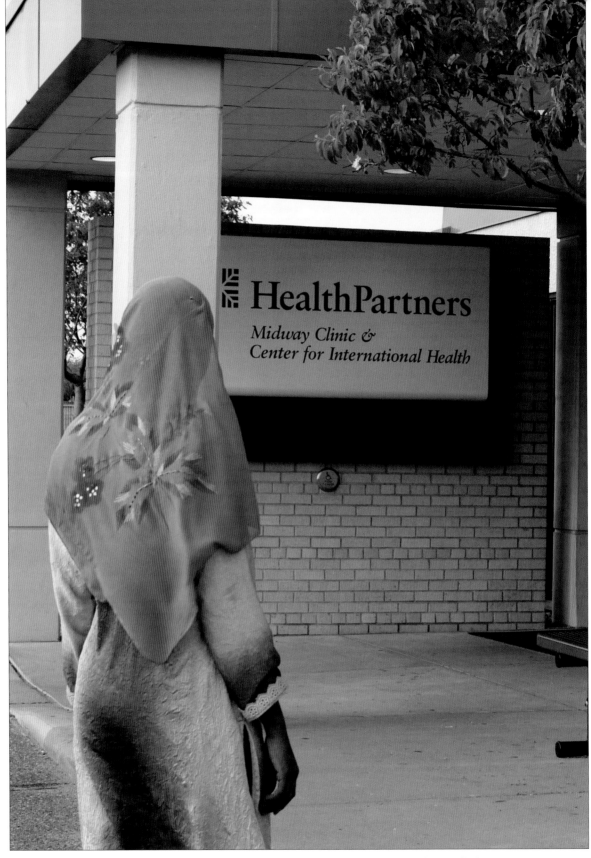

On May 1, 2006, the Center for International Health moved into its new home at 451 North Dunlap Street in St. Paul.

"my heart it is delicious"

transfer to the center so that he could see more immigrant patients during his residency training. He often marveled at the variety of illnesses we saw and the stories told by refugees from Somalia, Cambodia, Liberia, Vietnam, and Russia—stories of escape, torture, starvation, and loss of family as well as stories of survival and courage. As he listened to them, I could see the kindness in his eyes and the assurance in his voice as he offered healing. As his supervising physician, I could see that he did not need my mentoring on the principles of cross-cultural care; he embodied them already.

Physicians and patients throughout the world cross many cultures in health care. In this first decade of the twenty-first century, at least 185 million people worldwide live outside their countries of birth, up from 80 million three decades ago. Most health-care providers are practicing immigrant medicine to one degree or another. They want to improve the health of all of their patients, but it can be particularly challenging with recent immigrants, many of whom arrive from less-developed countries and with more infectious diseases, including intestinal parasites, hepatitis B, and tuberculosis. Protocols for screening new arrivals can be complex; physicians must be aware of differences in disease patterns by race and ethnicity, as well as by country of origin. Management of diseases heard of only in medical school can be difficult to remember.

Bridging the chasm of culture is a tall order, one that brings out the best and the worst in medicine. Every day in hospitals and clinics around the world, physicians struggle to provide high-quality health care to new immigrants whose health-care belief systems are often different. Personal capacity, training, and skills to reach across cultural chasms are often inadequate to prepare us for the changing demographics of our patient populations. Physicians-in-training acknowledge this feeling of lack of preparation in cross-cultural health care. They associate their greatest source of dissatisfaction with their patients' understanding of prevention and management of chronic disease. Patients feel even more lost, dissatisfied with both their care and the lack of compassion.

Why do some health-care systems create barriers and others reach out to communities in need? What is it that makes some health-care workers racist and others sympathetic to patients who are so radically different in their health-care goals and understanding? How do we help others to care? And, assuming the best—that we *do* care—how do we share that knowledge? "The secret lies in getting people to care about someone or something that is happening across the world from them," says one of my medical-school ethics professors. Dr. Paul Farmer of Harvard University has passionately stated, "The idea that some lives matter less is the root of all that's wrong with the world." Adds the physicist Virchow, "Medical education does not exist to provide students with a way to make a living, but to ensure the health of the community."

Because the world is at our doorstep, health-care systems must be redesigned to focus not on the provider or the source of payment, but on the patients, whether they are Haitian, Vietnamese, Ukrainian, or Mexican. There are many national and international examples of effective health-care delivery for immigrants, including those clinics and hospitals that hire providers who reflect the communities served. They also link mental-health providers and midwives to primary-care clinics and use professional interpreters, social work/case management staff, and community-health workers. The story of the Center for International Health is one of many such clinics around the country.

Over the years I have recognized personal core values that have helped me be clear in my purpose and passionate in my advocacy. Those core values include global health equity, respect, trustworthiness, cultural humility, and compassion. Physicians and other health-care providers must be knowledgeable regarding innovative ways to reduce health disparities for migrants. We should be advocates for change in this regard. Global health equity should be a fundamental goal of health care.

Cultural humility is another positive quality for clinicians dealing with any patient, but particularly those patients from different healing traditions. I am constantly struck by the danger of any modern drugs, as life-saving as they can be, and by the power of traditional healing methods used for centuries. Plant compounds used for centuries in China are now a key resource in the fight against malaria worldwide. Potato poultices are cheaper than microwave hot packs for my Russian patients with knee pain. Red yeast rice has been acknowledged as an alternative for treatment of high cholesterol.

Ultimately, however, it is through the stories of our patients' lives—lives that we are privileged to hold in our hands and hearts for a few moments, in an examination room or across a makeshift wooden table at a refugee camp clinic—that we may come closest to reaching across the cultural chasm to heal those who are suffering. This book is filled with such stories: about lives torn apart by war and oppression, about people who move by choice or under duress, about people who reinvent the American dream every day.

In *Tragedy in Paradise: A Country Doctor in Laos,* a friend of my father's and my mentor, Dr. Charles Weldon, describes working with the Hmong and training the first Hmong female nurses and medics. One of those medics broke his graduation certificate out of its frame and sewed it in his daughter's jacket before they fled Laos across the Mekong River. His certificate helped prove his refugee status. That young daughter is now a Minnesota state legislator, Mee Moua. The world has come to America, as our neighbors, co-workers, colleagues, and patients. And if we knew their stories, we would be amazed.

Although 99.3 percent of Americans are immigrants or the children of immigrants, America receives its recent arrivals with mixed feelings, citing drains on the economy and cross-cultural differences. Yet a 2005 Harvard Medical School study found that health-care expenditures for U.S. immigrants were approximately 55 percent less than those of U.S.-born residents. And although immigrants accounted for 10 percent of the U.S. population in 1998, they accounted for only 8 percent of all U.S. health-care costs.

Respect for the richness of my patients' culture, religion, and country of origin, as well as for the strength it takes to leave one's homeland, has created powerful bonds for me with my patients. They teach me every day about cultural humility, compassion, and courage in the face of overwhelming adversity. They remind me of the inadequacies of our medical

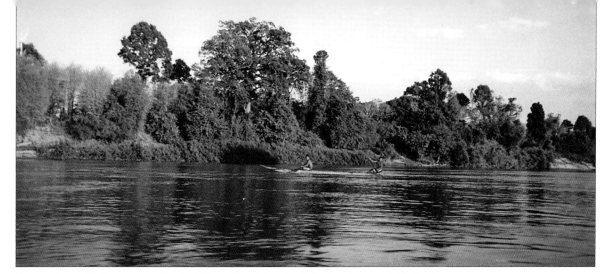

Hmong refugees fled Laos by crossing the Mekong River (above) to find refuge in camps in Thailand.

knowledge, and they challenge me to examine my own cultural biases. They help me gain perspective on American lifestyles and priorities as industrialized societies struggle with epidemics of obesity, diabetes, and heart disease. They make me dream again of one day working internationally.

My hope is that their stories, told so eloquently by Billie Young, will touch the hearts of ordinary Americans, of medical administrators, health insurance leaders, health systems experts, public health providers, and practicing clinicians. The good news is that young doctors and nurses are eager to learn, to travel the world from Laos to Uganda to Rwanda to deliver medical care where it's most needed. They come home transformed by what they have seen and determined to make a difference, to "walk the fine line between advocacy and outrage" as exemplified by Dr. Paul Farmer in Peru and Haiti, Albert Schweitzer in Africa, Dr. Tom Dooley and Karen Olness in Laos, Drs. Kathie Culhane-Pera and Neal Holtan in Minnesota, and Dr. Elizabeth Barnett in Boston.

And by Mrinal Patnaik in a small village in rural India.

Mrinal is now applying for a hematology-oncology fellowship at the best programs in the country, sparked in part by his knowledge of the bleeding caused by many tropical snake bites. He was offered a prestigious chief residency at the University of Minnesota but he turned it down, eager to return to India after his fellowship. Says Mrinal: "I am an academic and interested in research, but my passion is really what you are doing here at the Center for International Health every day: clinical care of patients."

While on a recent trip home for his brother's wedding in Mumbai, Mrinal took his mother to see the village where he had spent a year caring for its people. His compassion for them was well remembered; the entire village turned out to greet him. "Look!" said his mother from the passenger seat of the car. There, on the side of the check dam, was written "The Dr. Mrinal Patnaik Dam."

I am humbled by the tapestry that weaves the world together and deeply grateful to my parents, my family, my mentors, and my patients for the joy and privilege of sharing that tapestry which is life.

Patricia F. Walker, M.D., DTM&H
MEDICAL DIRECTOR
Center for International Health

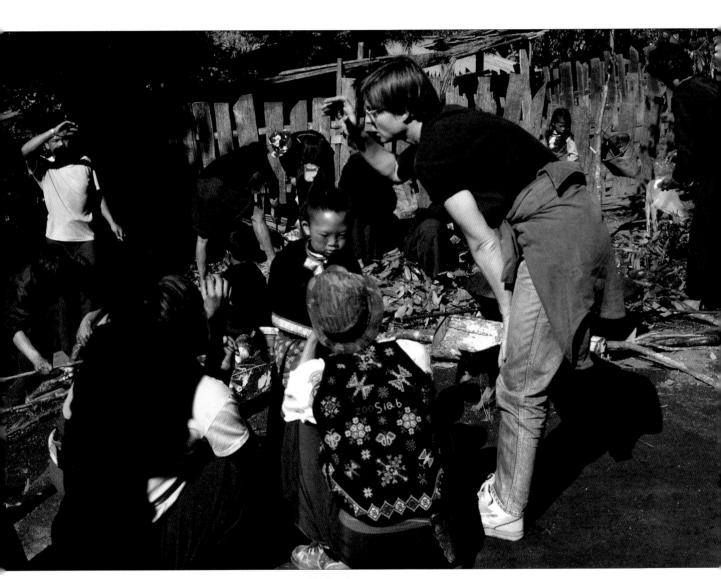

Dr. Kathleen Culhane-Pera at work in a Hmong village in Thailand.

prologue: lost in translation

IN THE EARLY 1980s, most physicians in the United States served a clientele whose backgrounds were much like their own. In the Upper Midwest, and in Minnesota particularly, doctors treated patients who had emigrated from Scandinavia, Germany, and the British Isles, as well as descendants of the old-stock New England families who had settled the region four generations earlier. Only rarely did Minnesota doctors encounter a patient like Mai.[1]

Mai was a one-week-old Hmong girl whose parents brought her to the International Clinic at St. Paul–Ramsey Medical Center. The newborn had a fever. The doctor who saw the baby immediately considered that Mai had bacterial meningitis, an inflammation of the brain and spinal cord that could have started in her lungs or her urinary system, or with exposure to strep infection. Unlike viral meningitis, which is not serious, bacterial meningitis is life-threatening. Survivors often suffer severe neurological complications, such as hearing or vision loss, learning disabilities, or seizures. Mai's doctor wanted to do an immediate septic workup to diagnose and treat her infection.

Through an interpreter, Mai's parents listened carefully as the physician explained

that their baby probably had meningitis, might not survive the night, and, if she did, would likely die within twenty-four hours without treatment. The doctor further explained that the septic workup involved three lab tests, each requiring a needle puncture: one to draw blood from her arm, a second to draw fluid from her spine, and a third to draw urine from her bladder.

Mai's parents, Hmong people from the hill country of Laos, were aghast at what the doctor proposed to do to their daughter. Hmong traditions strongly discourage the puncturing of holes in the body. The Hmong also believe that the body has a finite supply of blood that can never be replenished once it is lost. Mai's father looked into his child's eyes. Despite her fever, she appeared to him to be alert and content. The doctors, however, were adamant that the tests were necessary, and so, after much discussion, Mai's parents reluctantly allowed the blood test, but refused to let the doctors do anything more.

The technician had difficulty drawing enough blood from Mai. He jabbed the needle into her arm three or four times as her parents watched and worried that she was being mistreated, if not tortured. The small

[1] The names of all patients have been changed to protect their privacy.

sample showed that her white blood cell count had risen to fifteen thousand in response to the infection; a normal range is five to ten thousand. The doctor now insisted on doing the spinal tap.

When Mai's parents again refused the test, the doctor told them that if they did not give permission they could be arrested. He explained that even though they were her parents, they had no right to deny Mai medical treatment. The doctor could even have Mai taken away from them. And if they refused treatment and she died, they could be put in jail. The doctor's threat of jail angered Mai's father, who believed that he and his wife were responsible parents. Besides, why would Americans want to imprison him? Hadn't his people lost their homes and risked their lives to help the United States fight the war in Vietnam? Hadn't they immigrated to America to be free and safe among their allies?

Mai's father and mother, though young, came from an independent culture. They were used to making their own decisions, medical and otherwise. They found it hard to accept that doctors and social workers would not allow them to decide how their daughter should be treated. So they resolved to act on their own. While Mai's health team talked among themselves, her mother and father scooped her up, raced down a flight of stairs, found their car in the parking lot, and drove immediately to the home of a Hmong shaman, a traditional healer.

The shaman examined Mai and said that, although she had been frightened, she was in no danger and would recover from her fever. The shaman performed a ritual to settle the baby's fright, and when it was over, Mai appeared more alert. Her parents felt that the shaman had treated them and their daughter much better than the doctor had. It was late when they finally returned home.

Back at the hospital, the staff were distraught at the family's departure. They feared that Mai was seriously ill and would probably die without immediate intervention. They were determined to keep her and all other infants from being victims of their parents' ignorance. So they called Child Protection Services and obtained a court order to allow them to do the tests they felt were in Mai's best interest. Her parents were asleep when police officers knocked on their door. The officers told them that they had to take Mai back to the hospital so the doctor could take care of her. The angry father no longer had any way to resist. Accompanied by the police, the parents returned with Mai to the hospital, where, over their objections, a lumbar puncture was performed on Mai. As it turned out, she did have meningitis, but it was viral, not bacterial. Mai required no treatment other than hospital observation for two days and was then sent home.

Other Hmong parents experienced almost identical incidents with their sick children at the hospital. In their close-knit community, word passed from family to family: "Don't go to those doctors because they will call the authorities and force your child to be tortured. That doctor said that our child would die and he didn't, so don't believe anything anyone tells you there." The skirmishes became what University of Minnesota bioethicist Dr. Steven Miles calls "the meningitis and spinal tap wars of the 1980s."

≈   ≈   ≈

THE FAMILY OF MRS. VANG, an elderly Hmong woman, brought her to the emergency room of St. Paul–Ramsey Medical Center, gravely ill from a hemorrhagic stroke. An aneurysm in a blood vessel in her brain had ruptured. Pressure was building from the blood that had seeped through the tissue to the back of her skull. If her swelling brain pressed against the spinal cord and cut off the blood supply— a likely event—Mrs. Vang would die.

A neurologist told the family that to save their mother, surgeons would have to perform a craniotomy—to remove a piece of her skull to relieve the pressure on her brain. Mrs. Vang's husband, sons, and daughters all crowded around her bed, listening carefully to the doctor's diagnosis and recommendation. Then they talked among themselves before telling the doctor no. They did not want their mother's head cut open.

The frustrated neurologist called in a colleague, Kathleen Culhane-Pera, for help. Dr. Culhane-Pera, a family practitioner with a master's in medical anthropology, had done field work in a Hmong village in Thailand. The neurologist asked her to "talk sense" to these people and convince them they were wrong. She brought Mrs. Vang's x-rays to her meeting with the family and carefully explained how the surgery offered the best hope for Mrs. Vang's survival. The family listened, conferred, and

again refused. The neurologist began shouting at them, insisting that if Mrs. Vang did not have the operation she would die.

In saying, "She will die," the neurologist had unwittingly placed what the Hmong believe was a curse on his patient. Spoken by a powerful individual, such words initiate a field of energy that can have long-term consequences. If a cursed person becomes ill, the one who did the cursing must publicly and ritually apologize so that the sick individual can recover. In this case, the neurologist was curt and dismissive and stormed out of the room.

The next individual to confront the Vangs was a neurosurgeon, who also explained the surgery to the family and told them that, if they gave their permission, he would be the one to perform the operation. The family told the neurosurgeon that they wanted to take their mother home and have a shaman conduct a healing ceremony. A deeply religious man, the neurosurgeon respected and understood their position of faith. "Take her home," he told the family. "If she's not better, and you want me to do the operation, come back and I will perform the surgery." He kept open the door that the neurologist had slammed shut.

Mrs. Vang's family carried her home on a stretcher and up the stairs to her second-floor bedroom. That night, they gathered in their living room in front of an altar the shaman assembled to perform his healing ceremony. Dr. Culhane-Pera, who was acquainted with the shaman, had been invited to join the family.

The shaman's task was to find where Mrs. Vang's soul had gone and bring it back to her. He began the ceremony by picking up a large knife from the altar, its point piercing a stick of incense and its handle wrapped in one of Mrs. Vang's shirts. He attempted to balance the knife on the rim of a bowl filled with water. As he worked, he chanted. He went on chanting until he divined that Mrs. Vang's soul had left her body to be reincarnated into the fetus of an animal. If he didn't bring her soul back before the fetus was born, she would die. The shaman went into a trance, riding a bench called the winged horse on his journey into the spirit world. His seemingly interminable chanting ended when the knife suddenly stopped its teetering and hung there on the rim of the bowl, perfectly balanced. It was after midnight when the healing ceremony concluded.

The next morning the family decided that, while Mrs. Vang's physical condition had not improved, she was much better spiritually. They were convinced that she would now survive the operation because her soul had been safely returned to her body. After loading her onto a stretcher, they carried her back to the hospital, where the neurosurgeon performed the life-saving craniotomy. Mrs. Vang recovered and was back in her home a few days later.

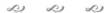

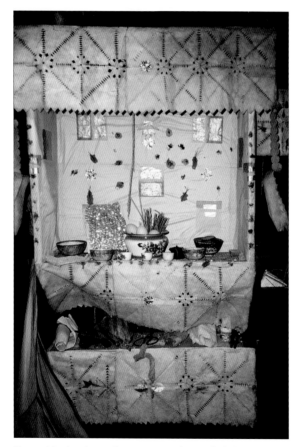

Pictured is the shaman's permanent altar, called the "Lub thaj neeb," which holds the shaman's tools. During shamanic ceremonies the shaman goes into a trance in order to connect himself with his helping spirits. In Mrs. Vang's case, it is probable that the shaman created a temporary altar for her specific healing ceremony. He would have located it below the family's altar on the spirit wall of the Vang home.

MRS. MOUA LEE had never been to a Western doctor. But when the goiter in her neck became so large that she had difficulty breathing, her sons brought her into the emergency room of St. Paul–Ramsey Medical Center. There, doctors found that a cyst on her thyroid had ruptured into an artery, which in turn had bled into the soft tissue of her trachea. She was suffocating. Mrs. Lee was rushed into the operating room, where doctors put a tube down her throat and into her trachea. Because her throat was so swollen, it was a difficult procedure, but the tube allowed her to breathe.

Doctors told Mrs. Lee's sons that she

needed an emergency tracheotomy—a hole in her neck through which they would remove the clotted blood, the thyroid gland, and the goiter. The hole itself would be temporary, they explained, and allow her to breathe while her upper airway healed. The operation sounded to Mrs. Lee's sons as if the doctors would be butchering their mother. They insisted that they needed several days to consider the doctors' advice before making a decision. This took place on a busy Friday afternoon.

By Monday, the hospital staff met again with Mrs. Lee's sons, who were still fearful of the tracheotomy. They wanted the doctors to remove the tube from their mother's throat. "This whole situation is dangerous," the doctors again explained. "Unless we put the hole in her neck, she won't be able to breathe. If we remove the tube, she won't be able to breathe on her own. But we can't leave the tube in there much longer, because the pressure of it is further damaging her trachea." Mrs. Lee's sons still wanted more time to think about it.

Mrs. Lee knew what she wanted. Her hands had to be tied to the sides of her hospital bed to keep her from yanking the tube out. Though she couldn't speak, her eyes and body language clearly communicated her feelings at the treatment she was receiving.

On Tuesday the sons announced their decision. They refused permission for the surgery and wanted the tube removed. The surgeon refused. If he removed the tube, he was not at all certain he would be able to put it back in. If he removed it and she

died, he would be committing murder. The stand-off between Mrs. Lee's sons and the doctors went to the hospital's biomedical ethics committee. A compromise was suggested. On Wednesday, five days after her arrival at the hospital, doctors would take Mrs. Lee to the operating room, put her under anesthesia, and look down her throat to ascertain the condition of her trachea. If it appeared to be all right, they would remove the tube but not perform a tracheotomy. The sons agreed.

However, when the doctors peered down Mrs. Lee's throat, they decided not to remove the tube. Her sons were outraged. If the tube were not removed that day, they declared, they would take their mother to another hospital. The ethics committee quickly met again and this time determined that the patient had the right to refuse treatment. A different surgeon was called, one who had no hesitation about removing the tube. He told the sons before they left the hospital with their mother that if she had trouble breathing again, they were welcome to bring her back and he would try to put the tube back in again. They agreed, took her home, and a shaman performed a healing ceremony for her.

Other than experiencing a very sore throat for a time, Mrs. Lee survived the removal of the tube.

∼ ∼ ∼

THE TWENTIETH CENTURY was the age of the uprooted. By the end of the millennium, 11.9 million people worldwide were refugees. An additional 23.6 million people were displaced from their homes. The United States alone has absorbed 1.5 million Vietnamese immigrants since 1975, as well as tens of thousands of Hmong, Ethiopian, Liberian, Somali, Russian, Sudanese, and Burmese refugees.

In the late 1970s and early 1980s, the thrust of international medicine was the work of travel clinics, where middle-class Americans came to get their malaria pills and shots before venturing into other, more hazardous parts of the world. According to Twin Cities public health physician Neal Holtan, there was no focus on the health of immigrants and refugees back then, no model of treatment or care.

Instead, a vast gulf of ethnicity, language, culture, and experience separated Western physicians from their immigrant patients. Despite the vaunted American health care system, they spoke past each other. Refugees who had survived extreme tortures found themselves facing not acceptance but misunderstanding. Disparities in health care dogged the daily lives of immigrants with inequities that, far too often, resulted in tragic outcomes.

Twenty-five years later, in hospital rooms and examining rooms throughout the United States, world views on medicine continue to collide. Immigrants still call into question the authority of Western

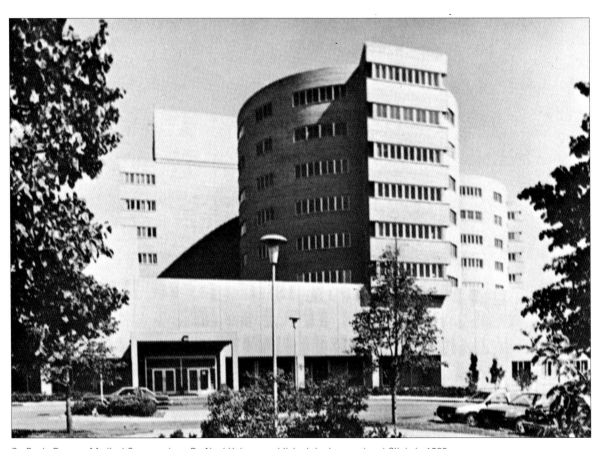

St. Paul–Ramsey Medical Center, where Dr. Neal Holtan established the International Clinic in 1980.

"my heart it is delicious"

doctors and their model of medical care—not because it fails them, but because it is not always open to their cultural concerns or to alternative methods of healing. Meanwhile, doctors who believe they are acting in their patients' best interests find, to their dismay and irritation, that their medical judgments are questioned. In the resulting standoff, the sick are not receiving care.

Back in the 1970s and 1980s, physicians at St. Paul–Ramsey Medical Center's International Clinic had their share of confrontations with St. Paul's newest immigrants. Since then, Minnesota has become home to the nation's largest concentration of refugees. Although Minnesota's population is still 90 percent white, the state has the country's highest number of Somali and Oromo and the second highest number of Hmong, most of them living in Minneapolis and St. Paul.

But it took a refugee crisis and a baker's dozen of Minnesotans responding to a call for help from the other side of the world to help develop a new concept and standard in immigrant medical care and bring it back home. The outcome was so unexpected, so radically different from most canons of Western medicine, that it went unrecognized for years—more an attitude or a sensibility than a tangible way to practice medicine.

Now called "culturally competent," this model of care grew out of the traumatic experiences of people caught between the grinding stones of war and dislocation. Many lives came together, lives and experiences more different from each other than can easily be imagined, to bring about this

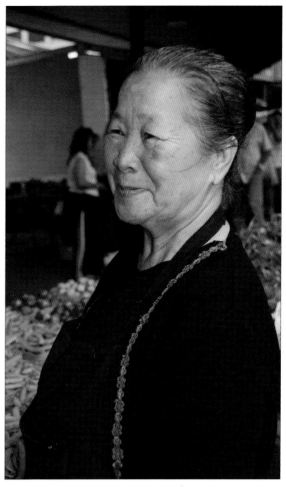

May Tho, a Hmong gardener resettled in St. Paul, sells her produce at the city's Saturday morning farmers' market.

new concept of health care and carry its message throughout the world.

Some practitioners extracted themselves from killing fields and prison camps. They came from Vietnam, Cambodia, Laos, Somalia, Kenya, and the Soviet Union. They included people as diverse as diplomats and the daughters of rice farmers. Though none could have imagined it at the time, they would one day meet in the cramped corridors of a St. Paul hospital, joined in a common cause of restoration—of overcoming cultural barriers to heal the sick and mend the broken.

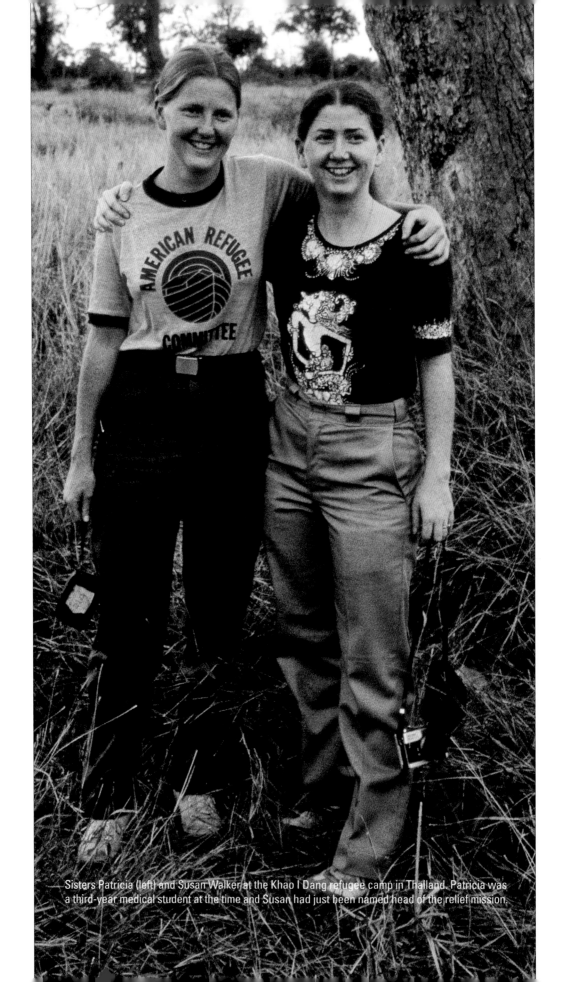

Sisters Patricia (left) and Susan Walker at the Khao I Dang refugee camp in Thailand. Patricia was a third-year medical student at the time and Susan had just been named head of the relief mission.

1: launching ARC

STANLEY BREEN WAS a juvenile delinquent, the son of Russian immigrants too old and too tired to cope with the new world into which their premature, youngest son had been born. As a result, "Trigger" Breen spent much of his childhood unsupervised on the streets of the old West Side of Chicago. In 1943, when he was thirteen, his mother died. Two years later, in the family conference that followed his father's funeral, a newly married sister, sixteen years his senior, reluctantly agreed to take Breen in.

His sister's generosity gave him a place to sleep but little else. He ran with a gang of boys who stole tires and robbed neighborhood stores. Though he managed to stay in high school, his grades dropped precipitously. What kept Breen in school was athletics. Though he wasn't tall, he had broad shoulders and arms strong enough to heave a basketball half the length of the court and, more often than not, drop it through the hoop.

After high school Breen enrolled in a junior college, but his heart wasn't in his studies. Joining the Air Force seemed like a better idea, and it was, until a horrific automobile accident in 1954 changed all of his plans. He spent months in the hospital and a year in a body cast recovering from multiple broken bones and internal injuries.

Breen was living in the basement of his sister's house in Chicago when he landed a job as a house parent at a treatment center for emotionally disturbed children. For the first time, he saw a way to give meaning to the life that had been salvaged from the auto accident. Breen would go to school and learn how to help kids who, in many ways, were just like him, kids he understood. He earned his sociology degree from Chicago's Roosevelt University and was directing a treatment center for emotionally disturbed children in Duluth when, in 1972, Wendell Anderson, the newly elected governor of Minnesota, asked Breen to become the human services official on his staff.

Events halfway around the world soon redefined Breen's job in the Minnesota capitol. The controversial Vietnam War was coming to an inconclusive end. North and South Vietnam signed the Paris Peace Accords on January 27, 1973, a treaty in which President Richard Nixon promised to provide military support to the South Vietnamese if the peace agreement were broken by the Communist North. Although Secretary of State Henry Kissinger and North Vietnam lead

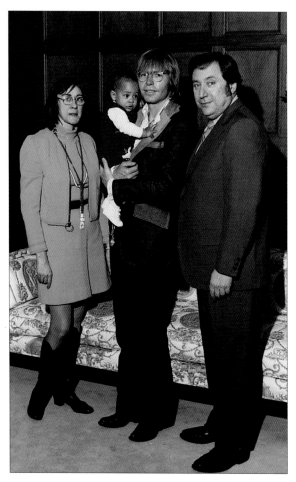

While working for Minnesota governor Wendell Anderson, Stanley Breen was instrumental in singer John Denver's adoption of a baby in 1975. From left: Breen's wife, Aviva, Denver with his just-adopted child, and Breen.

Nixon and Kissinger unenforceable. Power quickly shifted to the North and Saigon fell on April 30, 1975, unleashing a flood of refugees to America. Though the war ended for the United States, the turmoil was ongoing for the people of Laos, Cambodia, and South Vietnam.

The hill people of Laos, the Hmong, were at risk because they had supported the Americans in their secret war in that country. The CIA had recruited the Hmong in the 1960s to fight Vietnamese nationalists and Laotian Communists and to rescue downed U.S. pilots. By 1967 forty thousand Hmong were serving as ground troops for the CIA, ambushing Vietnamese supply lines on the Ho Chi Minh Trail and attacking Pathet Lao positions.

When U.S. airplanes dropped more than two million tons of bombs on northeast Laos, making it the most heavily bombed area in the world, the shelling disrupted village agricultural life to such an extent that Hmong families were forced to abandon their homes and move into the jungle. At the withdrawal of the Americans, the Pathet Lao government vowed to kill off the survivors, forcing the remaining Hmong to flee to refugee camps in Thailand. Almost all of the Hmong people who survived the Vietnam War and its aftermath had lost family members to imprisonment, torture, and murder by Thai soldiers.

The plight of the refugees was front-page news. The federal government appropriated money for refugee resettlement in the United States; Stan Breen took charge of Governor Anderson's ambitious refugee resettlement program in Minnesota. In 1977, when it appeared that sympathy for re-

negotiator Le Duc Tho won the 1973 Nobel Peace Prize for their efforts to end the fight, war continued in Vietnam as if no accords had been signed. Instead of withdrawing, China and the Soviet Union increased their support for the North Vietnamese.

America wanted out of the war in Southeast Asia. By December 1974, four months after Nixon resigned over the Watergate scandal, Congress had voted to cut off all military funding to the Saigon government, making the peace terms negotiated by fugees from Southeast Asia was flagging, Breen founded a thirty-state coalition of agencies and church groups that lobbied Congress to get assistance extended through 1979. Breen's name began to circulate among refugee-assistance communities as a man who could get things done.

Neal Ball

While Breen was working to resettle refugees in Minnesota, a Chicago businessman accepted an invitation that would shortly affect both of their lives. Neal Ball, vice president for public affairs of the American Hospital Supply Corporation, went to a fund-raiser held by his longtime friend, Enid Rivkin, widow of William Rivkin, U.S. ambassador to Luxembourg, Senegal, and Gambia. The event was held to raise money to resettle Vietnamese boat people fleeing the Communist takeover of Vietnam.

Ball had little interest in Vietnam refugees, but he couldn't say no to Mrs. Rivkin's appeal for help. He agreed to send a small monthly check to help support a refugee. A few months later he was astounded to receive a call from the U.S. State Department, telling him that the refugee he had sponsored would be arriving at Chicago's O'Hare Airport that coming Saturday and Ball should make plans to pick him up.

The brusque fifty-something businessman and a shy, self-effacing young Laotian laid eyes on each other for the first time at O'Hare. Phunguene Sananikone pressed his palms together and bowed as if in prayer to honor his sponsor. Ball wondered what he had gotten himself into. Though neither could speak the other's language, Ball mumbled a greeting, picked up Phunguene's bag, and led

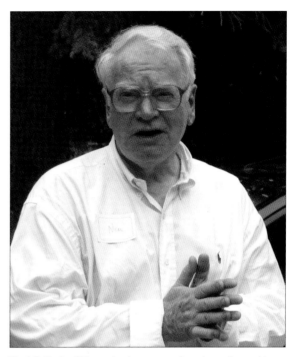

Neal Ball, the Chicago businessman who, almost by accident, became involved in the resettlement of refugees from Southeast Asia. Ball went on to found the American Refugee Committee, based in Minneapolis, which now works with displaced people throughout the world.

the way out of the airport. The next day he enrolled Phunguene in English classes.

With Phunguene living in his house, it was hard for Ball to avoid becoming involved in refugee resettlement. Within a few weeks, touched by Phunguene's story, Ball organized a network among his colleagues to sponsor refugees. One day, several months later, he observed that the typically reticent Phunguene had tears in his eyes. When Ball asked him what was wrong, the young man said, "Sometimes I think about my family." That was Ball's first inkling that Phunguene had relatives who also might be refugees. The young man's father had been a high-ranking judge under the old regime in Laos. Now Phunguene's parents, brothers, and sisters all were among his missing relatives.

Despite his efforts, he had been unable to turn up a single trace of his family.

How, Ball wondered, can a well-known family just disappear from a civilized country without someone knowing where they are? How can systems of government, of communication and transportation, of ordinary civility, break down to this extent?

Phunguene's situation was too much for the can-do Chicago business executive to accept. Ball resolved to go to Thailand himself and find the lost members of Phunguene's family. He took a week off from his work and, at his own expense and with the help of the New York–based International Rescue Committee, flew to Thailand's refugee camps, where, amazingly, he was able to locate one of Phunguene's brothers, his wife, and their children. At another camp he found a second brother and his family who, just days before, had swum the Mekong River to safety in Thailand, only to be forced back into Laos by Thai government soldiers. "I got a 'hold' placed on that return," Ball comments dryly. Though it took him five years, Ball arranged for eight members of Phunguene's family to immigrate to the United States.

What Ball saw in his whirlwind tour of the Thai refugee camps was that civilization, as he had always defined it, had indeed broken down. In desperate attempts to survive, people had abandoned homes and careers to hide from Communist soldiers intent on slaughtering every individual who was educated. The refugees navigated mine fields, swam rivers, and bartered with bandits in frantic bids to make it across a border to safety. Ball's eyes were opened. He came back from the camps convinced that some-

thing more than well-meaning individual efforts were required to deal with the refugee crisis. He decided to institutionalize his work.

Though he was employed full-time by the American Hospital Supply Corporation, Ball organized what he grandly called the American Refugee Committee. If he was intimidated by the fact that refugee work was traditionally carried out by bigger and better-funded agencies operating out of Geneva, Switzerland, and Washington, D.C., he didn't let on. Instead, he persuaded his friends to serve on his organization's board of directors, cajoled some nationally known figures—including Leonard Bernstein, Donald Rumsfeld, Adlai Stevenson, Admiral Elmo Zumwalt, and actor Ed Asner—to serve on an "advisory committee," and set about to find a director.

When he inquired around, the name of Stan Breen repeatedly came up. Ball was impressed by Breen's experience in the Minnesota governor's office, but it was more important to him that Breen's heart be in the right place. When the two men met, they found they had been cast from the same mold. Besides organization skills, what the pot-bellied, chain-smoking, fast-talking Breen had was passion. "Where did we all come from?" he asked. "Where did our grandfathers and great-grandfathers come from? Our nation was peopled by refugees."

Ball hired Breen, who, though not thrilled about the idea, agreed to move back to Chicago to head the new agency. Breen's wife, Aviva, and their four children had other ideas. Aviva was in law school and she and the children did not want to leave Minneapolis. So the American Refugee Committee opened its doors for business in donated space in the then dilapidated Flour Exchange Building in downtown Minneapolis. ARC's tiny fourth-floor office had two chairs, two desks, and a telephone. It was the spring of 1979.

Breen rented a warehouse to hold donations of clothes, food, and furniture for newly arriving refugees in the Twin Cities and hired Deb Anderson to run it. While she and Breen sat sharpening their pencils and waiting for the phone to ring, a series of events in Southeast Asia began converging to create the greatest refugee crisis since the end of World War II.

ARC's First Medical Teams

At first the crisis built slowly. The American Refugee Committee focused on finding sponsors for refugees from Laos and Vietnam and helping the sponsors find housing and jobs for the new arrivals. By the summer of 1979 the committee was grappling with a major bottleneck in resettling refugees. A local sponsor for a family would have everything ready to receive the new immigrants (an apartment, clothes, jobs) when, at the last minute, the sponsor would be told that the refugee family had been placed on a "medical hold." A medical hold meant that if any member of a family in a refugee camp slated for immigration to the United States was found to have an infectious disease, the whole family was automatically held back for one year before they could immigrate. This was discouraging to the local sponsors and demoralizing to the immigrant families.

Ball and Breen decided the solution was to do something about the health situation in the Thai refugee camps. Why not send their own medical team to look for infectious dis-

eases, check on the status of their immigrant families, and keep them healthy until they could board their flights to the United States? To recruit a medical team to go to Thailand, Breen needed additional help in his office.

Coincidentally, twenty-nine-year-old Karen Johnson was making the rounds of employment agencies, looking for work she considered "meaningful." She had left Augsburg Publishing after seven years, determined to find a job where she "could make a difference for people in the world." The agencies were of little help, but one evening she received a telephone call from a young man at an agency where she had interviewed. "Karen," he told her, "this is not through the agency, but I was at a DFL fund-raiser last night and I met someone I think you should call." That someone was Stan Breen. He hired Johnson on the spot and told her to find him a medical team to send to Thailand. It was September 1979.

A story in Twin Cities newspapers and Breen's appearance on local television spread the word that the fledgling American Refugee Committee was looking for volunteers to go on a short-term medical mission to Thailand. The office phone began to ring and within a week Johnson had selected her team. "I think picking people was my strength," she says. "I just chatted with them on the phone, asked why they wanted to do this, listened to the tone of their voices and their reasons. I had no time to check references. I only had time to make sure their medical licenses were genuine."

On October 8, 1979, three Twin Cities medical professionals, nurses DeAnn Rice

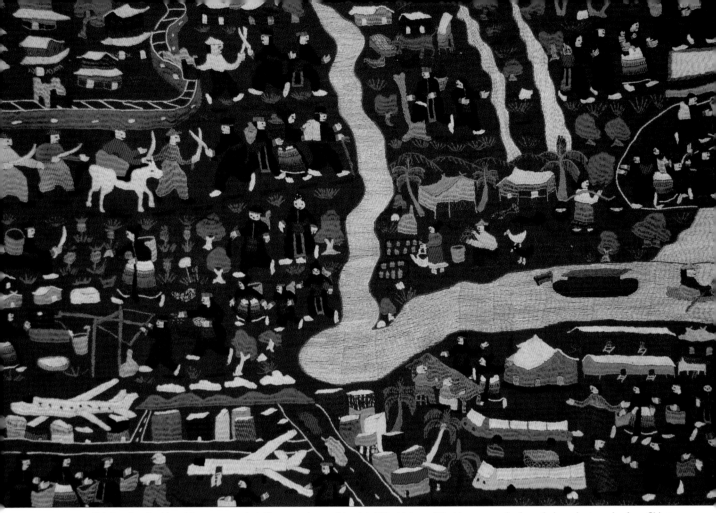

This hand-embroidered Hmong story cloth illustrates in exquisite detail the history of the Hmong people, from their ancient exodus from China to their flights out of Thailand to the United States. In the upper left are Chinese-style houses surrounded by the Great Wall of China. When the Hmong were driven out of China, one group fled east into Laos, a second group west to Burma. The story of those who fled into Laos is told on the right side of the cloth. When the Vietnam War broke out, bombing forced the people to flee across the flooded Mekong River to find sanctuary in the refugee camps in Thailand. Their arrival in the United States is pictured in the left bottom corner.

and Arnie Anderson, plus pediatrician Mace Goldfarb, and two physicians from California departed the United States for a refugee camp in Thailand under the auspices of the American Refugee Committee. Johnson had promised each of them $300 a month to help pay their living expenses and plane fare. At the time she made these promises, less than $7,000 was in the American Refugee Committee bank account.

Back in Chicago, Neal Ball was worrying about bigger things than money. The well-connected businessman had received a disturbing call from a friend, Henry Kamm, who was a *New York Times* correspondent. For months, Kamm had been following the aftermath of the invasion of Cambodia on Christmas Day 1978 by the Communist Vietnamese. He was one of the first in the Western press to realize that the steady advance by the Vietnamese would release Cambodians from the grip of Pol Pot's murderous four-year-old Khmer Rouge regime. The result, Kamm predicted, would be disastrous. In a lengthy, late-night phone call, Kamm told Ball, "You can't get enough help into there [Thailand]." Ball relayed Kamm's warning to Breen.

Upon their arrival in Thailand, the medical team sent Karen Johnson a telegram. "We are fine," it read. "We are among the Hmong." It was signed, "The ARC 5." United Nations representatives in Thailand had assigned the team to a Hmong refugee camp called Ban Vinai, in part because an evangelical organization already working there was having a terrible time making connections with the Hmong people. The health status at the camp was bad and the UN was, in effect, saying to the ARC 5, "Let's see if you can do any better."

The team from Minnesota soon found out what was wrong. The evangelical organization was more interested in proselytizing to the refugees than providing health care. Sensing this, the Hmong were reluctant to use its services. To induce the Hmong to come into their clinic, the evangelicals had resorted to using incentives. One of their tactics was to hand out Bibles to every individual who came to their clinic.

The Hmong were illiterate, in the Western sense; their language had been written down scarcely thirty years before. They had their own ancient, distinctive, and proud culture. Being a practical people, the Hmong accepted the Bibles offered to them and used the pages for toilet paper. "This is what happens when you don't think these things through," one of the Minnesotans dryly observed. After removing that roadblock, the five workers from the American Refugee Committee quickly built bridges to the Hmong community and began treating their many infectious diseases.

Two weeks from the day of their arrival in the camp, the team was hard at work treating

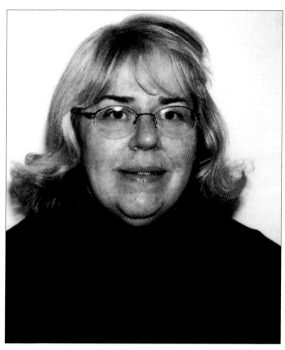

Karen Johnson Elshazly, whose search for meaningful work brought her to Stan Breen and the American Refugee Committee. Elshazly selected the participants for the first teams sent to Thailand. She joined ARC in 1979 as its third employee and is still there.

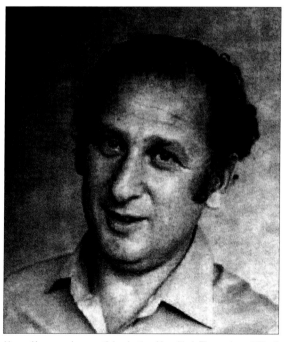

Henry Kamm, whose articles in the *New York Times* alerted Neal Ball to the impending refugee crisis in Cambodia and Thailand.

patients in Ban Vinai when word reached them that 750,000 desperate Cambodian refugees from the Pol Pot regime were, at that moment, pouring across the border into Thailand. Kamm's dire prediction had come true. In their tiny ARC office in Minneapolis, Breen turned to Johnson and said, "You did that first team. You know how to do it. So put together a second team for the Cambodian border."

Within three days, Johnson assembled a second medical team, this one made up of fifteen individuals: seven physicians (Daniel Susott, Neal Holtan, Steven Miles, Celeste Woodward, Lawrence Kaplan, Carol Juergens, Solomon Cutcher), six nurses (Barbara Huwe, Virginia Baresch Ascensao, Judy Rothen, Deborah Turk, Emilie Beck, Patricia Stuart), one paramedic who was also a second-year nursing student (John Lapakko); and a medical student (Pat Walker). To manage their relief mission in Thailand and serve as team director, Johnson signed up David Ziegenhagen, publisher of Minnesota's Sun Newspapers, who had been a deputy director of the Peace Corps in Thailand. Ziegenhagen left for Thailand a few days ahead of the medical team.

Neal Holtan, one of the physicians whom Johnson recruited, says Johnson had a sixth sense about people: "She could read a resume and tell if it was phony or not. She could talk to people on the phone and get more out of it than anyone else with a two-hour interview. She picked all the right people to go on these missions."

All of the ARC 15 volunteers set aside personal and professional commitments for their varying stints in the camps, some four weeks long, others several months. Holtan, a graduate of the University of Iowa's College of Medicine with a master's degree from the University of Minnesota School of Public Health, had just been hired at St. Paul–Ramsey Medical Center by director Bob Mulhausen. Mulhausen almost fired Holtan when he said that he was taking a leave to work in a Cambodian refugee camp.

Recalls nurse Barbara Huwe, "I checked it out with my husband and daughter and they both said go." Huwe, who had read about ARC's call for help, had been married just a year and had a nine-year-old daughter from a previous marriage. She had never traveled out of the United States.

The Walker Sisters

The news headlines about the crisis on the Cambodian-Thai border attracted the attention of Susan Walker, a writer for the *Minneapolis Finance and Commerce Daily News* who was about to enter law school. She had grown up in Thailand, one of five children of a U.S. pilot. She called her younger sister Pat, a third-year student at Mayo Medical School in Rochester, Minnesota, to alert her to what was happening in Thailand, adding that the American Refugee Committee of Minneapolis was organizing help. "You've got to go," Susan told Pat.

Hardly giving her sister's directive a second thought, Pat called Karen Johnson at the American Refugee Committee office. "I don't have a lot of clinical skills," Pat explained. "But I know Thailand, I speak Thai, and I could probably help with things like logistics."

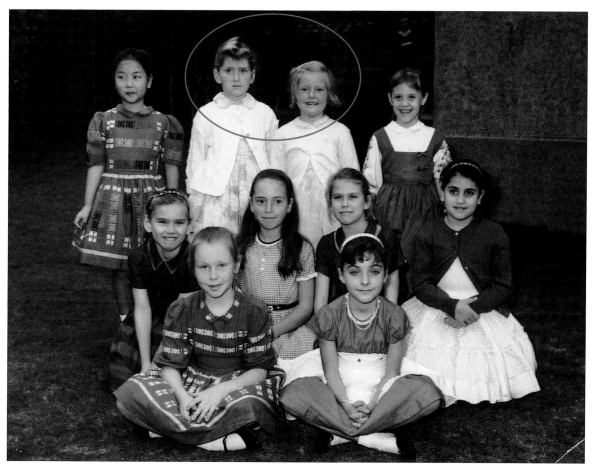

Susan and Pat Walker in 1959. Seven-year-old Susan (back row, second from left) and four-year-old Pat (back row, third from left) were living in Taipei, Taiwan, while their father flew planes in Vietnam, Laos, Cambodia, and Taiwan.

"You're on the team," Johnson told Pat. Only then did Pat ask her dean if she could go.

The Mayo Medical School was still new—Walker was in its fifth graduating class—and had never released students to do volunteer work overseas. Though the dean was reluctant to let her go, he eventually agreed to give her credit for two of the weeks she would spend in Thailand and let her make up the rest of her work.

Pat Walker was thrilled to be of help. The crisis in Thailand was afflicting a country she thought of as her first home. Born in

1955 in Taiwan, she had lived with her parents and four siblings in Bangkok, Thailand, until she was eleven. Her father, Frederick Walker, was chief pilot for Air America, the CIA's secret airline in southeast Asia. While the Vietnam War was under way, she was aware that her father did dangerous work for the airline—moving refugees, dropping rice to Hmong people living in the mountains, and flying in and out of tiny airstrips carved out of the jungle. She did not find out until later that he was involved in the United States' secret war in Laos.

Pat and her siblings also did not know that

their parents' marriage was in trouble. The Walkers' divorce came as a surprise to Pat and her brother and three sisters, as did the news that the girls were moving with their mother to Gulfport, Mississippi, where Pat's mother, Phyllis, had a married sister. (The girls' older brother was in the army and stationed in Germany. Their youngest brother was born in 1976, to Fred and his second wife, Sally Lee Chang Hwa, a Chinese woman who had grown up in Thailand.) "We felt as if we were stepping off the edge of the world," Pat remembers.

In a way, they were. They moved from an ethnically diverse city of a million people in Southeast Asia to a segregated town of 32,000 in the deep South of the United States. It was 1966, and busing for racial balance was under way. The racial tension profoundly affected Pat, who attended an all-white segregated junior high school. "Every single day after school, the black and white kids were fighting," she recalls. "I watched this and could not understand it. Why were they so mad at each other? Why did the white kids hate the black kids?"

Pat's second cultural shock was an educational one. She was three years ahead of her classmates at Bayou View Junior High School. "I was the only girl in the eighth grade to get straight A's," she remembers. "And I never studied. I was bored stiff." She and her sisters were critical of America and disdainful of what they believed to be the provincialism of Mississippians, most of whom didn't know where Thailand was. Pat's younger sister Elizabeth spent her first year in the United States eating her lunch in the school bathroom. "We felt lost," Pat remembers.

It was all the girls could do to wait until summer, when they would return to Thailand to live with their father. They spent four months a year with him, leaving school a week before it formally ended in the spring and returning a week after it started in the fall. That first summer, fifteen-year-old Susan memorized the passport numbers of twelve-year-old Pat, eleven-year-old Liz, and four-year-old Nancy as they flew, unaccompanied, to meet their father in Bangkok.

After Hurricane Camille devastated the Gulf Coast in 1969, Phyllis Walker decided to return with her daughters to her native Minnesota, where the rest of her family lived. The girls settled into the vastly different (and better) educational system in Minneapolis. That year, when she was fourteen, Pat learned more precisely what it was that her father did in Southeast Asia.

Early in his career, Fred Walker was one of the thirty-seven U.S. pilots who flew 682 secret sorties to drop supplies to the French during the battle at Dien Bien Phu in the spring of 1954. As chief pilot for Air America, it took Walker some time to figure out who he worked for. He and his fellow pilots simply referred to Air America as "the Customer." Walker knew that some of his flights were flown for the CIA, but he didn't learn until the early 1960s that the airline was owned by the agency. At that time, Air America was the world's largest airline. It was also the airline with the world's highest mortality rate.

As chief pilot, Walker was responsible for the safety and welfare of Air America's pilots. Because of the fighting going on in Vietnam and Laos, he did not permit his pilots to fly at night, requiring them to return to the Lao capital of

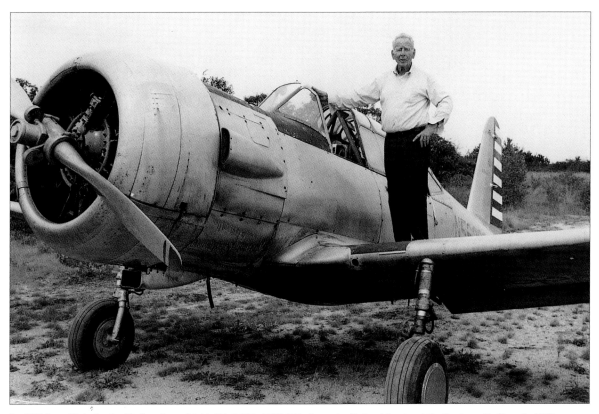

Fred Walker, chief pilot for Air America, with his World War II BT-13A plane, the *Vultee Vibrator*, at the Fryeburg Air Show in 1996.

Vientiane before sunset. Upcountry villages were falling to the Communists and downed pilots were in danger of being trapped. But one evening, two agents of "the Customer" who were strangers to Walker drove onto the airfield in Vientiane and asked to talk with him. The agents sat in the back of the car while Walker slid into the seat beside the driver. One of the men leaned over the seat and told him, "We want you to start flying at night."

Walker refused, but the agents weren't interested in his protests; they told him that the pilots had no choice but to begin flying night missions. Walker was a big man, six feet four, whose deep voice added to his commanding presence. When he realized that he was getting nowhere with the agents, he got out of the car, said, "I'm not

going to do it and that's final," slammed the door, and walked away. A few days later he was summoned to Air America's headquarters in Taipei, Taiwan, where the airline's president, Hugh Grundy, told Walker that the CIA owned the airline and that, yes, he *did* have to do what the agents at the airfield had told him to do.

The Walker children were avid followers of international news. When the Vietnam War ended with the defeat of South Vietnam and the departure of Americans from Saigon, they thought their father might be dead. They had not heard from him and had no way of knowing he had been evacuating refugees from Phnom Penh until Cambodia fell to the Communists on April 17. Walker had then gone on to Saigon to do the same

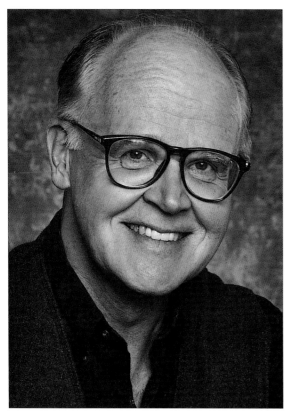

David Ziegenhagen, who went to Thailand to head ARC's refugee efforts on the Cambodian border until Susan Walker replaced him.

until South Vietnam fell on April 30. Fred Walker flew the last Air America plane out of Saigon on April 29, 1975.

"Until I started college, I was my father's daughter," Pat Walker remembers. "Dad told us stories of the North Vietnamese and Pathet Lao and how they would torture prisoners. I grew up in a house that was rabidly anti-Communist. My father's U.S. home in Maine had the flag of the former Soviet Union wrapped around a rubber floor mat so that when we walked into the house we would step on it. That is where I was, philosophically, until I went to college and started to realize there were other sides to the story. For many Vietnamese, it was a war of liberation that had started with the French occupation."

Back to Thailand

Twenty-three-year-old Pat Walker headed to Thailand with the ARC 15 on November 9, 1979, riding in seats donated by Western Airlines. When they landed in San Francisco, they found that their overseas flight, on which they also had donated seats, was canceled. The mission might have ended then had a frantic Breen not reached an acquaintance in Florida, who agreed to put the flights to Bangkok on his credit card. Breen did not tell his volunteers that not only was he unable to repay the debt before the bill came due, he also had no funds to bring them home.

Breen did not have long to worry. Media reports of the Cambodian disaster spurred Minnesotans into contributing. On November 12, *Time* magazine published a cover story headlined "Deathwatch: Cambodia." Wrote the reporter: "Stumbling on reed-thin legs through the high elephant grass that grows along the frontier, they [refugees] form a grisly cavalcade of specters, wrapped in black rags. Many are in the last stages of malnutrition. In 1975 the country had a population of approximately 8 million; as many as 4 million Cambodians have died since then." The cover photograph showed a mother holding her starving baby.

"We would come to work every morning, and there were so many envelopes with money and checks under the door that we had trouble opening it," Karen Johnson remembers. "We would literally have to shove the door to get it opened." Hundreds of people called every day to see how they could help.

Susan Walker, who was following reports on her sister Pat and the medical team in the *Minneapolis Tribune,* began volunteering at the ARC office after work hours. One Monday night, two and a half weeks after the ARC 15's departure, she was greeted at the ARC office by Johnson, who was holding a telegram from team director David Ziegenhagen in Bangkok. It read: "Million refugees at border. Absolute humanitarian crisis. Cannot handle this alone. Send Susan Walker." Johnson handed her the telegram and said, "You'll be the deputy director. Can you leave on Saturday?"

When Susan Walker arrived in Bangkok on December 3, 1979, another note from Ziegenhagen was waiting for her. "Dear Susan," it began, "I was not at the airport to meet you because I am at the hospital with your sister Pat, who was bitten by a rabid dog and is getting rabies shots. Be back soon. Please read attached briefing paper and get up to speed because my wife is divorcing me and I'm leaving. You are now the director."

Walker was twenty-six years old.

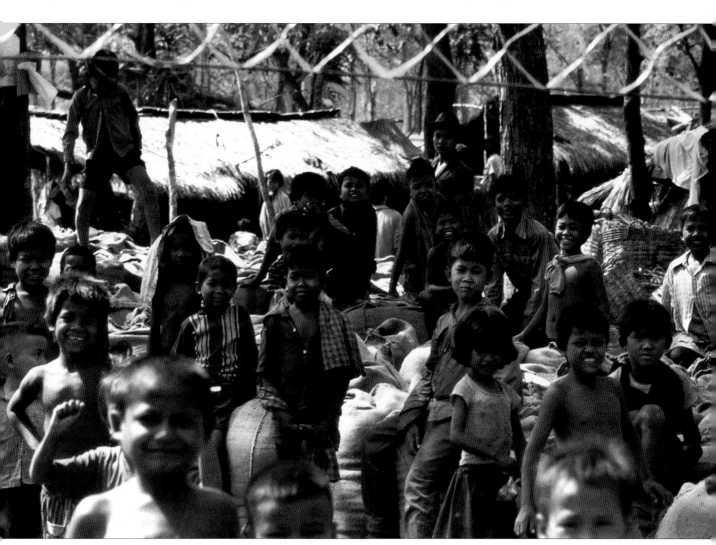

Cambodian children at the Ban Nong Samet refugee camp located on the Thai-Cambodian border.

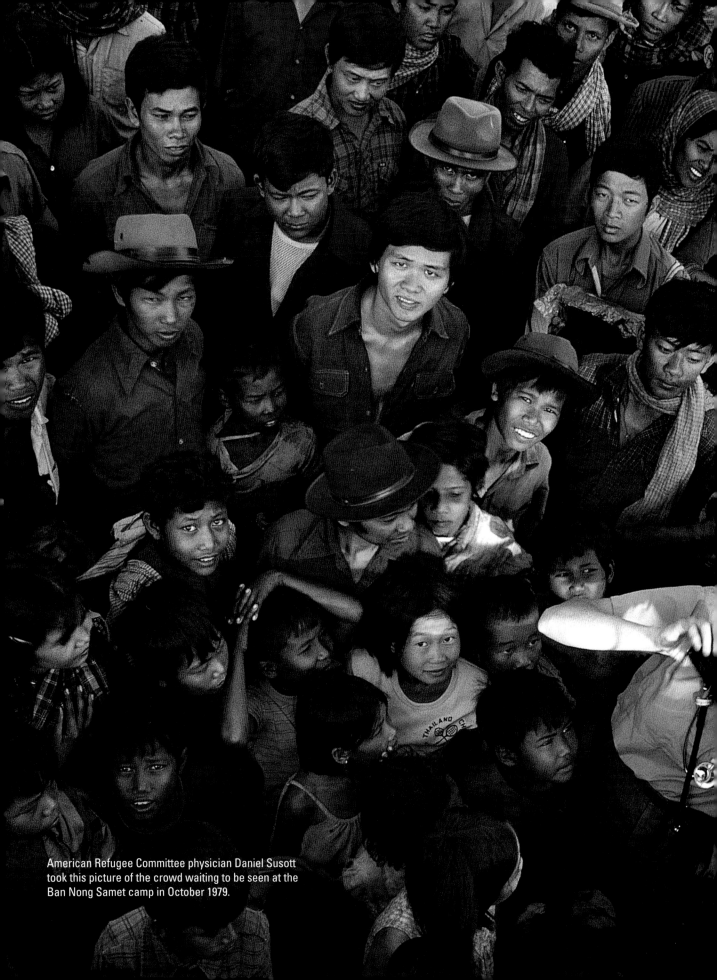

American Refugee Committee physician Daniel Susott took this picture of the crowd waiting to be seen at the Ban Nong Samet camp in October 1979.

2: culture shock in Thailand

THE TEMPERATURE WAS 100 degrees and rising when the ARC 15 arrived in Thailand in late November 1979. The first camp the team went to was Sa Kaeo, where five physicians and nurses from Germany had been struggling to care for five thousand desperately ill people. The camp was set in a soggy rice field on land that could not be drained, and the first rains of the monsoon had turned the camp into a sea of mud. Malnourished refugees, too weak to turn themselves over, lay face down in the mud and drowned. Emaciated babies died in their mothers' arms. More people died outside than inside the hospital, a bamboo-framed shelter that was open on all sides, with a roof of blue plastic tarps covering a dirt floor. Whenever it rained, health-care workers poked sticks at the sagging tarps to keep them from collapsing on their patients. They were not always successful. Nurses frequently found lifeless patients lying in shallow pools of water. As many as forty people died in a single night.

After one day at Sa Kaeo, the ARC 15 moved to Ban Nong Samet, a refugee camp on the Cambodian-Thai border. Their clinic consisted of three examining rooms inside a bamboo-framed building with a thatched roof. The volunteers, led by Minneapolis gastroenterologist Lawrence Kaplan, saw four hundred patients a day: case after case of malaria, anemia, malnutrition, tuberculosis, and diarrhea, Dr. Kaplan's specialty. Some patients had deep hip abscesses, the result of injecting themselves with antimalarial medication they had bought on the black market. Because water and food often ran out by noon, doctors had to turn away mothers with starving babies. Dr. Dan Susott could do little more for a twelve-year-old orphan boy (who looked to be about seven) than to pin a tiny vial of vitamins inside his tattered shirt and wrap a towel about his thin frame. When the boy bowed and pressed his hands together to thank the doctor, Susott began sobbing while his nurse, herself in tears, held shut the door of their hut.

At night, small-arms fire reverberated through the camp, evidence of the ongoing fighting between the Vietnamese and the Khmer Rouge (the "Red Cambodians") and the Khmer Serei (the "Free Cambodians"). Khmer Serei soldiers, boys and girls who looked to be teenagers, strutted around the camp carrying battered M-16 and AK-47 rifles.

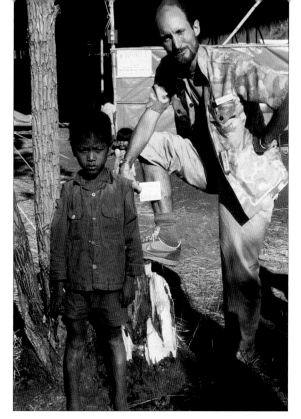

The rabid dog that bit Pat Walker at the Khao I Dang refugee camp also bit four others, including Dr. Daniel Susott, above, before it was shot by Thai soldiers.

ARC Ward 1

Concerned about the limitations of the Ban Nong Samet camp, and faced with the daunting task of coping with thousands more refugees who were fleeing Cambodia, Thai officials built a new camp about seven miles from the border. The Khao I Dang camp was constructed in two weeks. With help from Thai and refugee workers, the ARC 15 set up the first hospital at Khao I Dang in two days. "We were at Khao I Dang on the day it opened," Pat Walker recalls. "We were the only hospital ready to accept patients on day one."

Walker made a sign identifying the facility as "ARC Ward 1, Staffed by Kampuchean Volunteers and the American Refugee Committee." As at Sa Kaeo, the hospital was made of bamboo poles supporting a plastic

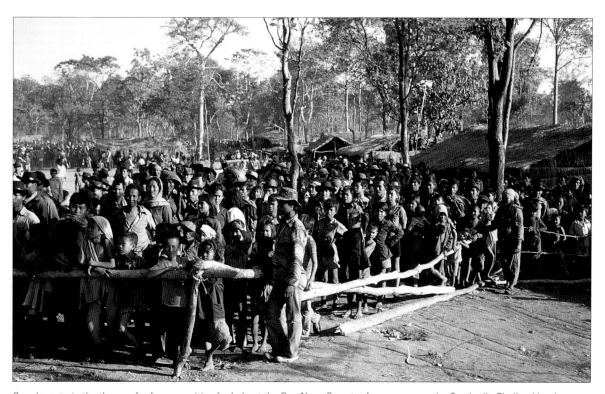

Guards restrain the throng of refugees waiting for help at the Ban Nong Samet refugee camp on the Cambodia-Thailand border.

tarp over a dirt floor. There were 110 "beds"—sheets of plywood on metal frames, each covered with a woven mat. The hospital without walls offered its patients no privacy.

ARC Ward 1 had eighty-seven admissions in the first five hours. Patients waited all day in long lines to get in, including "mothers with their babies standing in the hot sun for hours, waiting for someone to see them," recalls nurse Barbara Huwe. Patients of all ages came in, carried into the hospital on homemade stretchers or in the arms of family. Because everyone who was admitted was dehydrated, doctors and nurses automatically stuck needles into their arms and hung IV fluid bottles on plastic strings from the ceiling. Entire families slept on a single bed.

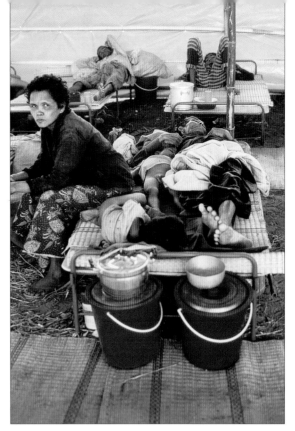

Entire families slept on the board beds in Khao I Dang hospital. The red buckets at the foot of one of the beds are for food.

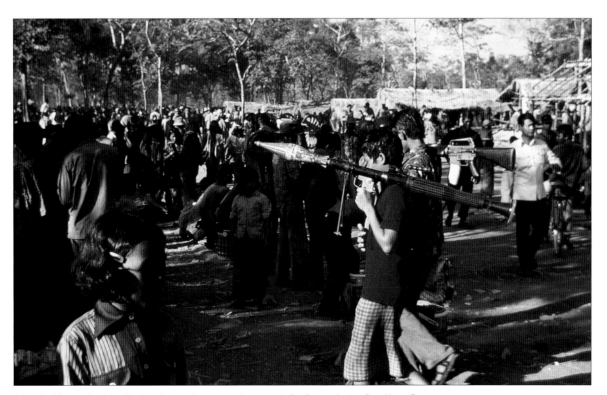

A boy holding a shoulder-fired rocket walks among the crowd of refugees in the Ban Nong Samet camp.

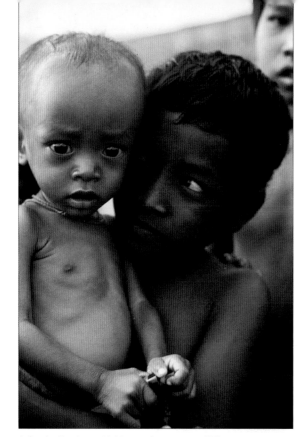

A Cambodian boy with his starving younger sibling.

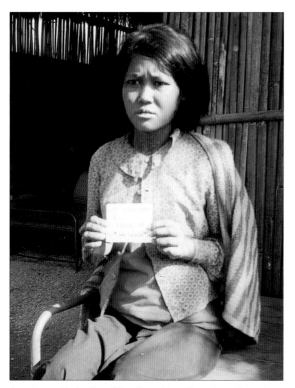

A patient suffering from "Casal's necklace," a rash on the neck and face caused by a niacin deficiency.

Trucks brought the refugees from the border and dropped them in a field within the camp. Because the Minnesota team was desperate for translators, Huwe and Steve Miles, a twenty-nine-year-old medical resident, began meeting the trucks and pulling aside any refugees who spoke even a little French or English.

One refugee who clambered off a truck was a Madam Hauey, described by Miles as an "absolutely brilliant" woman who had run the midwife hospital in Phnom Penh before the fall of Cambodia and who spoke perfect French. Since Miles also spoke French, the two quickly formed a bond. They were working together in the camp when Miles noted a man suffering from a catatonic depression. "It was classic waxy catatonia," he remembers. "I had read about it, but I had never seen it before. You could put this man's limbs in any position and he would stay there. I asked Madam Hauey, 'What is this?' She replied, 'Much sadness is the cause of this.'"

Diseases rarely seen in the West were the norm in Thailand. Severe malnutrition was often the underlying culprit, especially in children, whose distended stomachs indicated kwashiorkor, a condition caused by a lack of protein in their diet. Vitamin deficiency, present in almost every refugee who came to the camp, made beriberi, pellagra, leprosy, and similar diseases commonplace. Beriberi, caused by a thiamine deficiency, has two forms: dry beriberi, which results in such severe nerve damage to hands and feet that standing or walking is impossible, and wet beriberi, which causes congestive heart failure. Camp physicians were puzzled to see heart failure, a disease of the elderly, in young refugees. To their surprise, their young patients got better when they began taking B vitamins.

"I saw things I would never see in the States," Walker says. Pellagra, an often fatal disease related to niacin deficiency, causes a skin eruption around the neck called "Casal's necklace." "If you show that to the average physician in the United States," she says, "they may think it is sun sensitivity." When she went to the latrines, she would see parasitic roundworms two feet long and as thick as her little finger that people had passed in their stools. Sometimes she would see children pulling the worms, called *Ascaris*, out of their noses. Instead of being repulsed, Walker found the camp hospital

experience fascinating and it cemented her growing interest in tropical medicine.

Acutely aware of the limitations of being a medical student among nurses and physicians and fearful of being a burden to them, Walker had read two textbooks on tropical medicine, cover to cover, before she boarded the plane for Thailand. One disease she read about was Madura foot, an essentially untreatable fungal infection that occurs in people who walk barefoot over rice fields. The disease slowly deforms the foot as it infects the fatty tissues and the bone. One day, when Steve Miles was puzzling over a patient's misshapen and painful foot, he called Walker over to take a look. She said excitedly, "I think that's Madura foot."

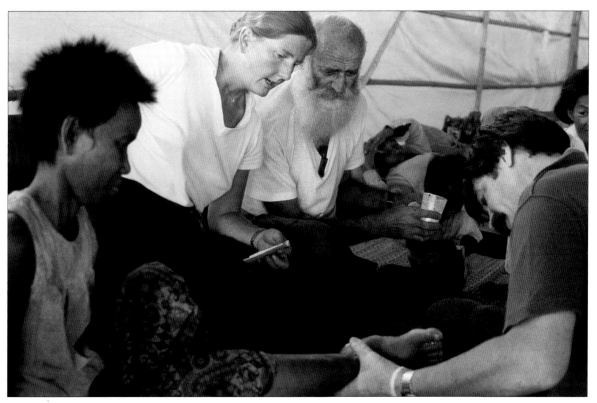

Medical student Pat Walker, Dr. Solomon Cutcher (center), and paramedic John Lapakko examine a Cambodian woman with leprosy. She had developed a foot ulcer because she was unable to feel her feet as she walked barefoot across the fields.

Reading her textbooks had paid off. "Now I felt as if I had really contributed something," she says.

Worried that she might be asked to do procedures in Thailand she had not yet learned back in Minnesota, Walker had also brought with her *Manuals of Medical Therapeutics*, a standard textbook series used by medical students. Early one morning, as she walked by the labor and delivery ward run by the French nongovernmental organization called Doctors Without Borders, a physician took her aside and said, "You're closer to your medical school education than I am. I want you to sew up this episiotomy for me."

Walker knew that it was unheard of to do episiotomies in Cambodia. For whatever reason, midwives there just did not do the procedure. Yet here was a woman whose doctor had cut her vaginal opening to ease a difficult delivery and now he was unsure how to close it up. If he didn't close the wound, it could become infected or the woman could hemorrhage.

Walker had watched many episiotomies before, but she had never performed nor repaired one. Nevertheless, she studied the illustrations in her manual and sewed up the wound. She thought she had done a decent job, but had doubts the next day. She asked Dr. Dan Susott to check on the patient, saying, "I'm nervous I might have done something wrong." She had indeed. Her suturing was good, but she had used nonabsorbent thread. "I had to go back and undo what I had done and then redo it," Walker recalls. "That poor woman! And I was so mad at that physician. Why had he put me in a position to do something beyond my expertise? Then I realized that he might not have sewn her up at all, which would have been worse."

Soon Walker was delivering babies and assisting with appendectomies. She even learned how to pull teeth. Family practitioner Solomon Cutcher, whose white hair and beard made him look like Santa Claus, first taught her how to inject lidocaine into a

Dr. Solomon Cutcher removes an abscessed tooth from refugee Yong Yuth Banrith. Cutcher is assisted by Cambodian refugee physician Haing Ngor.

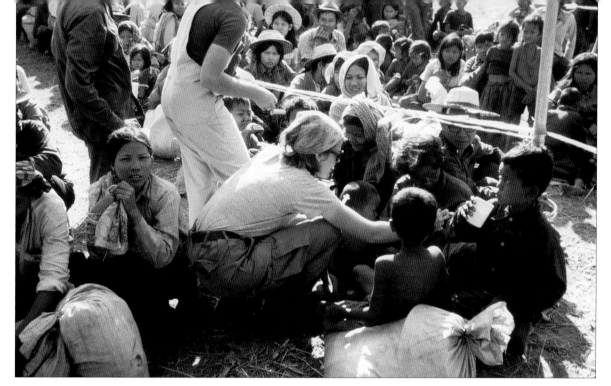

ARC nurse Barb Huwe triages patients at Khao I Dang who arrived by bus from the Ban Nong Samet camp on the Thai-Cambodian border.

patient's jaw, then showed her how to pull the rotting teeth.

Susan Walker, meanwhile, was busy establishing the American Refugee Committee as one of the most respected medical NGOs in Thailand. She was responsible for all aspects of management, policy development, and relations with local and international authorities. She supervised the ARC staff, which in six short months grew from fifteen volunteers in two camps to fifty-two staff in five-plus camps, as well as several hundred local staff who operated medical programs in the Lao, Hmong, Vietnamese, and Cambodian refugee camps. She also oversaw a mobile medical team for Affected Thai Villages. What began as Susan Walker's commitment of six to twelve months with ARC would turn into fifteen years of living and working in Thailand.

Training the Refugees

When the Minnesotans first arrived, they focused on saving lives and alleviating suffer-

ing. But when the camp population swelled to 87,000 refugees within six weeks, and then to 135,000, Steve Miles and his fourteen colleagues realized that their priorities had to change. The refugees were a traumatized people who, if merely given assistance and then left to dwell on the disaster that had overtaken them, would languish. They had to be helped to help themselves.

As the ARC 15 looked out over the expanse of needy people in the camp, they acknowledged that the foreign medical staff, no matter how large it grew, could never take care of everyone. They also knew that it was irresponsible for them to provide services for a short time and then leave without finding a way to sustain those services. The answer, they decided, was to leverage their expertise by training the Cambodians to be medics.

Already overworked, the nurses nevertheless wanted to find a way to teach the refugees how to be medical assistants and

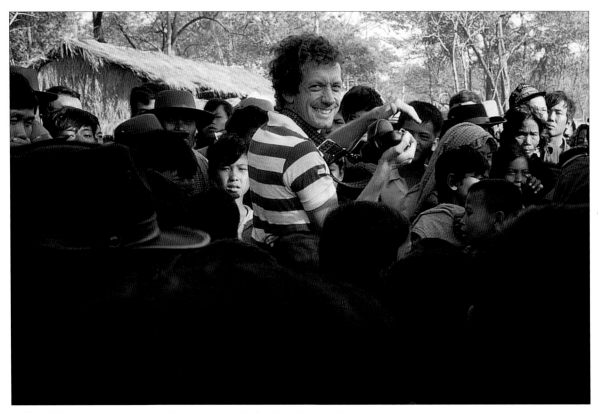
Dr. Steve Miles surrounded by Cambodian refugees at the Ban Nong Samet refugee camp.

midwives, as well as interpreters. "We already had a list of drugs set up by the UN and World Health Organization," Miles says. "We just had to establish treatment protocols. For example, a high fever with no cough would be presumed to be malaria. So give those patients the malaria treatment."

Miles was convinced that if they mobilized the refugees into a program where they could help themselves and gain some skills, they would also gain hope for the future. The "philosophy of care" statement he wrote stated that the American Refugee Committee would provide a level of care that could be taught, learned, and practiced inside Cambodia and Thailand. The program he put into effect in that first camp not only changed the way the ARC 15 provided care,

but it also established the long-term philosophy of the American Refugee Committee. As Miles puts it, "What we see now is the echo of how the relationship between the relief system and the relief service population changed at that time. Every time we trusted the refugees, the program bore fruit."

Miles resumed going to the camp perimeter every morning to meet the truckloads of new refugees and enroll anyone who spoke English in courses that would turn them into health-care workers. Barbara Huwe remembers Miles as a gentle teacher, extremely well read. "He had a strong sense of justice, of right and wrong," she says. "It pervaded his being. I think he was really the leader of our group—not the dynamic one, but the most reasonable, stable person."

"my heart it is delicious"

The first course trained refugees to be medics who could triage incoming patients—to determine who was sickest and needed treatment first. Another course trained refugees as nurses, birth attendants, and community health workers who could find the sickest people in the camp and bring them into the hospital.

The Cambodians responded with enthusiasm to the opportunity to help each other. In fact, so many men between the ages of twenty-one and thirty applied that the ARC 15 had to establish a quota so that women could get training as well. In the beginning the students followed the doctors around the hospital and, assisted by an interpreter, listened to their explanations. Later the staff built a bamboo classroom with a blackboard and benches and taught a detailed curriculum. "The incentive for the students was the opportunity to learn, to go to school," Pat Walker remembers. "Everyone was envious of those who got in. As they graduated, we gave each one a diploma that we made up, had printed in the town, and gave out at a ceremony. Graduates were so proud of those certificates that they framed them and hung them on the walls of their huts."

Walker was astonished at the variety of people she met in the camp and annoyed when the American media described the refugees as simple peasants. The prima ballerina of the Cambodian national dance theater was there, as was the nation's leading sculptor, who asked Walker, "What can I sculpt to thank America for this help?" There were college students and professionals of all kinds who had managed to stay alive through nearly half a decade of starvation, slaughter, land mines, and civil

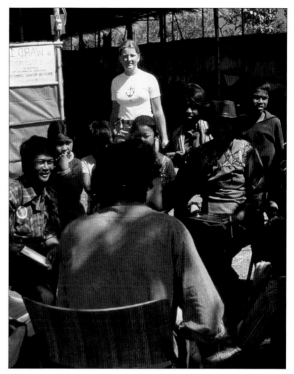
Dr. Larry Kaplan conducts a class for aspiring medics. Yong Yuth Banrith is on the far left; Pat Walker is in the background.

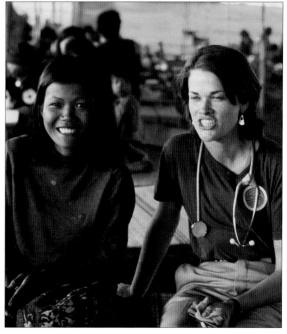
Nurse Barb Huwe and a volunteer Cambodian staff member in ARC Ward 1 at the Khao I Dang refugee camp in Thailand.

war. They were the improbable and heroic survivors of a Cambodian holocaust.

Haing Ngor and Yong Yuth Banrith

One day a thin young man walked into the camp hospital and asked how he could help. He said he was a physician from Phnom Penh who had been a prisoner in Cambodia. After coming into power in April 1975, the Pol Pot regime had killed all but forty-eight of Cambodia's six hundred doctors. This particular physician had lost every member of his family, including his wife. He alone had survived four years of torture by lying about his background, pretending he could not read, hiding his glasses and watch, and burying his medical texts and instruments in the ground.

The refugee doctor went to work immediately. He treated patients, translated for them, and became friends with Pat and Susan Walker, Steve Miles, and other members of the ARC team. His name was Haing Ngor, and he would later become known to the world when he won an Academy Award for portraying *New York Times* photographer Dith Pran in *The Killing Fields*.

Other Cambodian refugees came into ARC Ward 1 to help as translators. Yong Yuth Banrith arrived within the first week of the hospital's opening. "I was a university student in history in Phnom Penh when the Khmer Rouge took over," he told the camp doctors. "I speak some English. How can I help you?" Banrith was neatly dressed in a shirt, pants, and shoes, unusual in that setting. At first glance the staff thought Banrith had been luckier than most. His face was round and plump, and he did not appear to be as malnourished as other refugees. Then

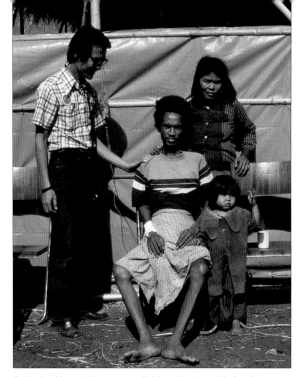

Dr. Haing Ngor with an appendicitis patient and his family.

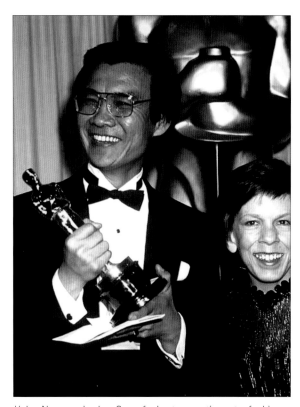

Haing Ngor received an Oscar for best supporting actor for his role in *The Killing Fields,* presented by Linda Hunt on March 25, 1984. Twelve years later, Ngor was found shot to death outside his home in Los Angeles on February 25, 1996. Police said the forty-five-year old actor was killed by an unknown assailant.

they realized that his body was swollen from the edema of kwashiorkor.

Though he was just twenty-five, Banrith looked at the world through the eyes of a much older man. "He had lost forty-three members of his extended family and clearly looked as if he had been through hell," recalls Walker. Adds Huwe, "Everybody's story was

tal translators, lived in the medical ward. Dr. Susott often found them, exhausted, in the small hours of the morning, "huddled like puppies on a bare board bed."

When Walker had night duty, doing rounds of patients by flashlight, Banrith kept her company. As the two talked and compared their student experiences, they became

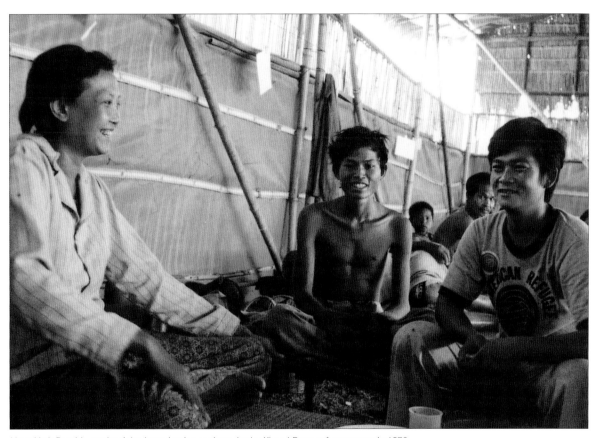

Yong Yuth Banrith, on the right, interviewing patients in the Khao I Dang refugee camp in 1979.

equally horrific. They had all seen people murdered and had survived by eating insects and rats and whatever they could get."

Banrith worked nonstop at the hospital as an interpreter. When the day shift left, he stayed on to help the person on night call. He and Haing Ngor, along with other hospi-

friends. "We bought Banrith a guitar and it turned out he had been a fan of American popular music," she says. "We would sit outside the ward and he would play John Denver's ballads—'Take Me Home, Country Roads' and other songs. We needed to defuse a lot, establish normalcy, find some joy in the day."

"Normalcy" was hard to come by. The Khao I Dang camp was enclosed with barbed wire and patrolled by armed guards. No one could enter or leave without permission. Except for one or two volunteers who stayed to do rounds, foreign medical personnel were not allowed in the camp overnight. Thai government officials, aware of the dangers surrounding the volunteers, trucked the ARC 15 off to lodging in the village of Aranyaprathet every night, a forty-five-minute trip each way. When the foreigners were gone, the guards terrorized the refugees with extortion and rape.

Yet as the days and weeks passed, smiles replaced cries. Children's kites rose in the hot air above the camp while toy cars, ingeniously constructed of old metal cans and soda bottles, zipped by underfoot. "The strength of the Cambodians was a recurrent theme at our meetings over dinner each night—their eagerness to help on the ward, to learn English, their quickness to say thank you for every pill or shot dispensed," Walker remembers. "For many, it was the first time in years that food was plentiful and that they could sleep through the night without waking for fear the Khmer Rouge or Vietnamese were upon them."

Roots of Cross-Cultural Care

As international authorities struggled to manage the torrent of refugees, a classification

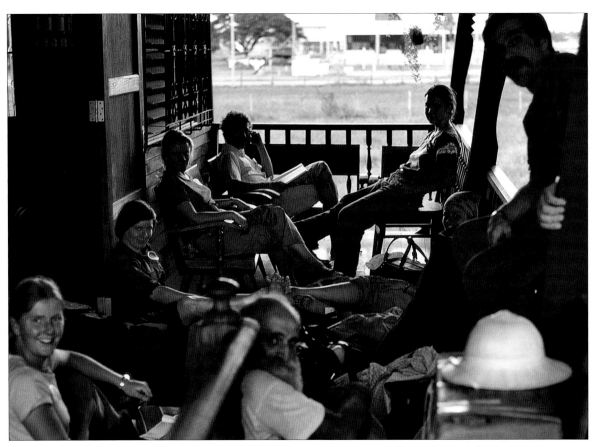

ARC team members relax on the porch of their inn in the village of Aranyaprathet. Clockwise from left: Pat Walker, Emilie Beck, Deborah Turk, Steve Miles, Carol Juergens, Barbara Huwe, John Lapakko, and Solomon Cutcher.

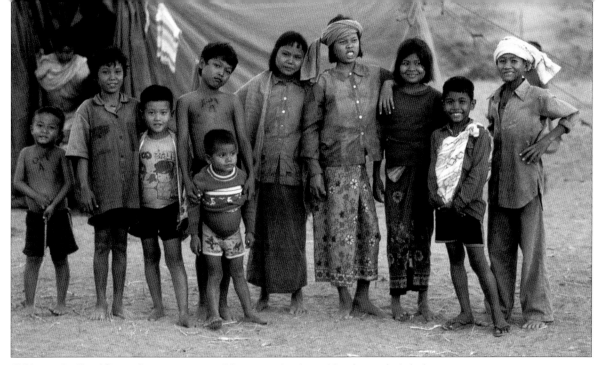

Children at the Khao I Dang refugee camp were quick to respond to the positive changes in their circumstances.

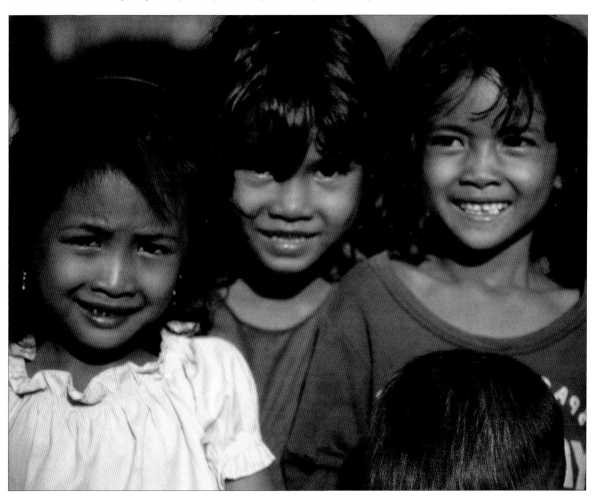

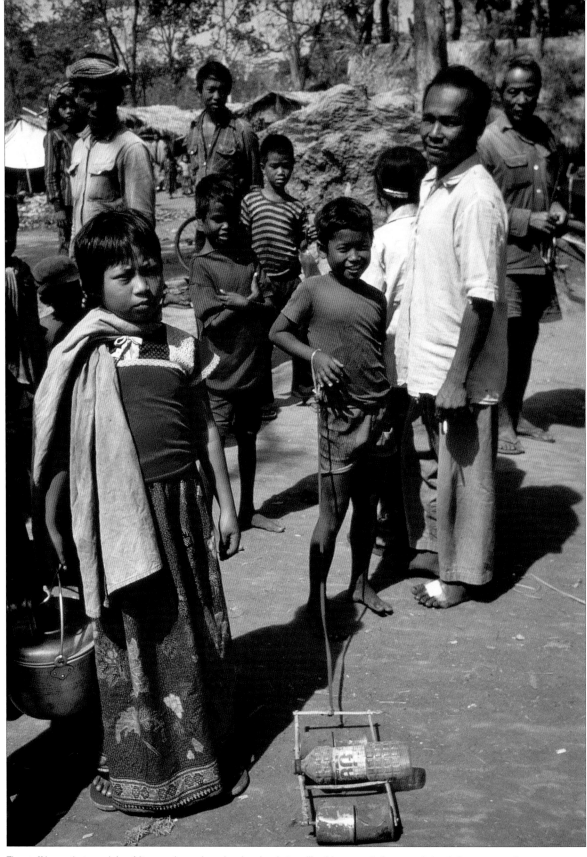

The staff knew that people's spirits were improving when handmade toys like this car made from a soda bottle began appearing.

"my heart it is delicious"

of the many border camps gradually emerged. Khao I Dang camp was the only one managed by the United Nations' High Commission on Refugees, and its residents were given all the rights that refugees were due, including eligibility for asylum, immigration to other countries, and assistance in maintaining minimal nutritional and health standards. All other camps were managed by the UN's Border Relief Operations and supported by various nongovernmental organizations, or NGOs, including the American Refugee Committee of Minnesota. Residents of these camps were not classified as refugees but as displaced persons, and therefore were not eligible for any of the rights due to refugees, such as the opportunity to relocate to another country.

The distinction between refugee and displaced person was arbitrary, a matter of timing that reflected the date on which a person showed up on the border. Those who fled earlier went to Khao I Dang and were classified as refugees; those who came later were displaced persons. The camps for displaced persons were legally under Thai government control, which handed over their management to various resistance factions—a guaranteed prescription for violence.

Because the Cambodian refugee crisis was so catastrophic, it changed the character of the NGOs. It appeared to Steve Miles and others that the NGOs had essentially been forced to reinvent their organizations. Previous NGOs had consisted largely of missionary-type organizations that offered services in a hierarchical, paternalistic manner. But the youthful leaders of the new NGOs, who had grown up during the U.S. civil rights movement,

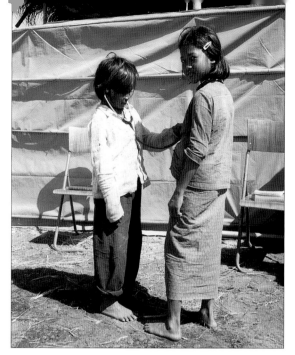

Two little girls play at being doctors and nurses at the Khao I Dang camp. Children's laughter began to lift everyone's spirits.

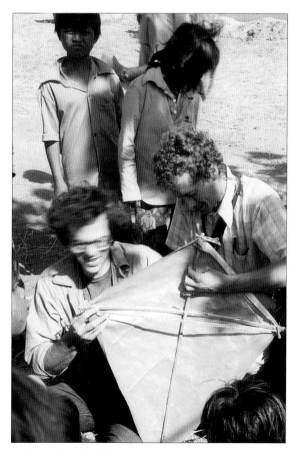

Dr. Steve Miles (right) and Dr. Larry Kaplan makes kites with Cambodian children.

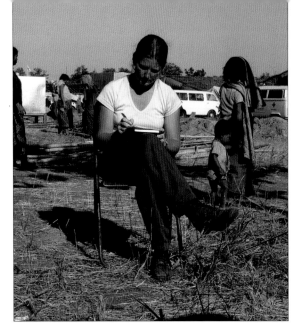
Pat Walker steals a moment to write letters home.

were open to new forms of grass-roots organizing. Miles remembers that they were "less doctrinaire, less evangelical, and more interested in seeing how we could work together to blend cultures and create peer relationships." Though they could not know it at the time, these NGO leaders were forging the philosophy that would become the foundation of cross-cultural medicine.

Looking back on the experience, Neal Holtan marvels at how the little American Refugee Committee, which sent its unprepared people to Southeast Asia on a shoestring, had managed to do one of the best jobs of caring for the sick in the region. He attributes its success to the fact that ARC had no government or religious affiliation. "We were more neutral than the Red Cross; we were not nationalistic like the Europeans, who were really very ethnocentric: 'You are either Swiss or you are not.' The French are like that too. All of a sudden our director, Susan Walker, was getting elected chair of the CCSDPT—the Committee Concerned for Services to Displaced Persons in Thailand steering committee, head of all the voluntary organizations in Thailand—be-

cause we were not threatening. I think that helped the NGOs exist and prosper."

Lessons Learned

Too soon, the ARC 15's stint came to an end. The doctors and nurses needed to get back to their families and practices; Pat Walker had to return to medical school. But those few weeks forever changed the lives of the team and the focus of ARC itself.

For Dr. Neal Holtan, the refugee experience was revelatory on two counts: not only in how others reacted to the overwhelming disease and senseless deaths they saw, but in how he himself reacted. One team member, Holtan recalls, was a "Minnesota golden-boy-type" who had never been out of the state. On their first night in Ban Nong Samet, the young man curled up in a sleeping bag next to Holtan. When Holtan got up the next morning to go to the camp hospital, the young man remained behind, apparently asleep. For the rest of the day, Holtan looked for his coworker to show up at the hospital, but he never appeared. When Holtan returned in the evening, the young man was still in his sleeping bag.

"I think it just overwhelmed him," Holtan says. "It wasn't as if he had some kind of underlying mental illness. Mentally he was well before he went to the camp. He just could not cope with it. It took him three days to adjust and then he was fine. That made me more respectful of culture shock."

Holtan knew that his own response was lacking when he saw nurses Ginny Baresch and DeAnn Rice begin caring for long lines of children with scabies, a skin infection that ran rampant in the camp. Holtan thought the nurses were "ridiculous to concentrate on scabies when one hundred feet away were these other kids who were dying of meningitis, tuberculosis, and stuff that we could cure if we tried." Why were the nurses and other volunteers wasting time on treating skin diseases, head lice, and rotting teeth, regardless of how many patients queued up to have those minor problems tended to?

"Well, I was totally off-base and did not understand it," Holtan confesses. "They were not just getting rid of the scabies; they were affecting the kid, the family, their nutritional status, finding ones that had other really bad problems and referring them, getting them fresh clothes. Think of clean clothes in that camp!" He had been making every decision a matter of life and death, thinking only of treating the disease, while the nurses were treating the whole person. "It was a whole new way of looking at things," he admits.

For Barbara Huwe, "culture shock was far worse for me coming back to the States than it had been going over." On the return layover in Hawaii, she spent a few hours at the home of her sister and brother-in-law. "I opened her refrigerator and it was full of food, and I couldn't believe it. It was Christmas time and the papers and TV were full of ads for gifts, useless material things that looked just gross to me. The camp situation was bad, but I could deal with it. Coming back to the U.S. was worse. The shock lasted longer."

Huwe was so affected by her experience that when she got home she quit her nursing job to find work that was more in line with what she had done in the camp in Thailand. "Public health seemed like the nearest thing [to the camp experience] because the Hmong

people were starting to [immigrate to the Twin Cities], so I went to work for St. Paul–Ramsey County Public Health," she says. She also convinced friends to join her family in sponsoring a Hmong immigrant family.

"Barbara Huwe came home from Thailand and said, 'We need to do something and get it going,'" Holtan observes. "Those missions we went on did more for Minnesota than for the refugees. They provided the nucleus of leaders in [our local] health-care system. . . . Minnesota gained far more than it gave."

For ARC founder Neal Ball, the lesson learned from the experience was a simple one: "Don't be afraid to offer help just because the problems are large."

While some members of the ARC teams may have expected to return from the refugee camps to the lives they had known before, most found that an impossibility. The Twin Cities, like many of the workers themselves, were on the cusp of dramatic change. Immigrants from Southeast Asia were settling in Minneapolis and St. Paul in ever increasing numbers. Despite the brevity of their camp experiences, the workers identified with the refugees' traumas. They now regarded their health-care practices through more critical eyes. Cultural and language barriers to heath care, situations that they had once ignored, now seemed like problems that demanded solutions.

In finding those solutions, some of them would transform a tiny clinic in St. Paul into an internationally recognized model of how to provide culturally sensitive health care to refugees and immigrants. None of them would imagine the difficulties that lay ahead.

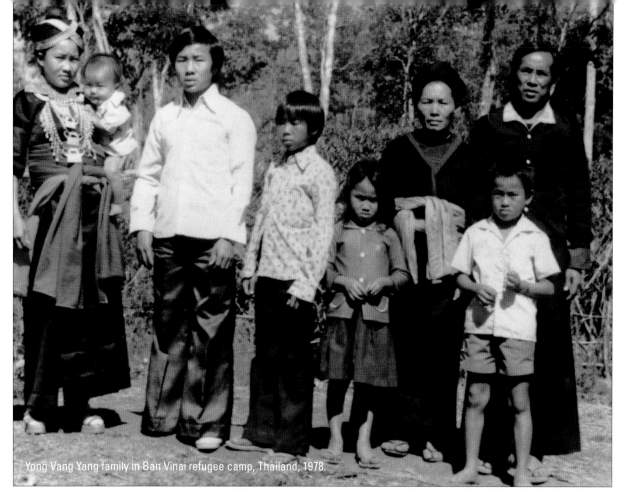

Yong Vang Yang family in Ban Vinai refugee camp, Thailand, 1978.

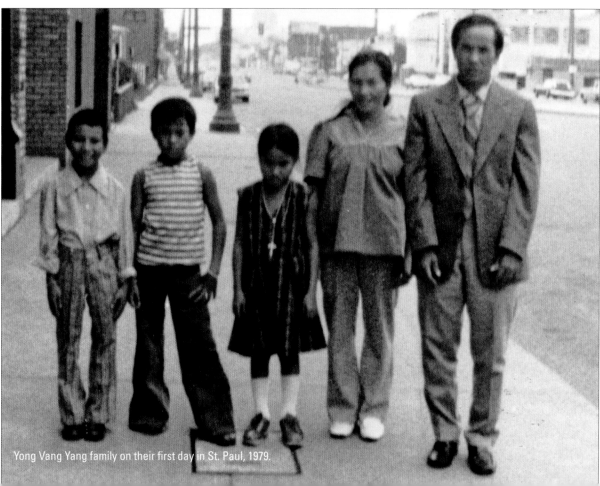

Yong Vang Yang family on their first day in St. Paul, 1979.

3: the international clinic debuts

WHEN INTERNIST NEAL HOLTAN resumed working at St. Paul–Ramsey Medical Center following his weeks at Khao I Dang refugee camp, he saw its approach to immigrant medicine with fresh eyes. The city's newest immigrants, hundreds of Hmong from Thai refugee camps, came to the hospital seeking basic health care. But instead of slipping seamlessly into the Western model of medicine, they were clogging up the system like willow roots infiltrating water lines.

"When a specialty clinic such as cardiology had a Vietnamese, Laotian, or Hmong patient, the clinic just ground to a halt," Holtan recalls. Without a common language or interpreters, no one could understand anyone else. As simple a matter as calling a patient from the waiting room into the examining room became a production. Nurses and nursing assistants could not pronounce the patients' names. They did not know which name came first and which came last. Several patients would simultaneously answer to a name because they shared similar or same names. "It was a big fiasco, hard on everyone, doctors and patients," Holtan remembers.

Hmong children, who learned English faster than their parents, were pressed into service as interpreters in examining rooms. White-coated doctors, stethoscopes dangling around their necks, found themselves counting on youngsters who had barely mastered "Sam I Am" or "Dick and Jane" to translate diagnoses and

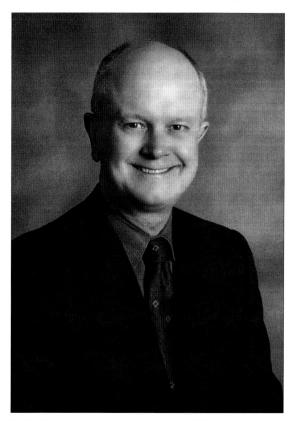

Dr. Neal Holtan, founder of the International Clinic, later called the Center for International Health. Holtan is medical director and tuberculosis physician at the St. Paul–Ramsey County Department of Public Health.

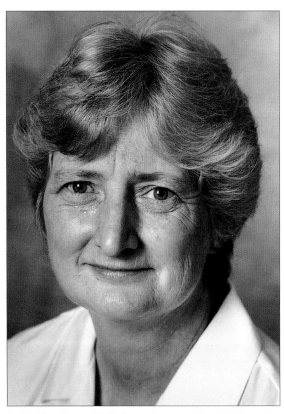

Pediatrician Carolyn McKay's experience working with the rural poor in Nicaragua gave her insight into the plight of Hmong immigrants new to the Twin Cities.

treatment instructions. Many physicians could not (and would not) address matters they wanted to talk about with their patients if their only means of communication was through the filter of a patient's child. Parents too were often reluctant to share personal health matters with physicians when their children were the language brokers.

Language and Cultural Barriers

"If you cannot communicate with the patients," Holtan says, "it is like practicing veterinary medicine." Without a medical history from the patient, a doctor has to rely on observation and laboratory results to make a diagnosis. Cultural differences made some diagnoses tougher to make than others. Many Hmong, for example,

came to the hospital complaining of severe abdominal pain. Doctors responded with their usual battery of diagnostic exams: CT scans requiring the patient to drink barium, endoscopies requiring the patient to swallow a camera at the end of a tube, even exploratory surgery. But more often than not, the tests came back negative; the baffled doctors could find nothing wrong. What they failed to understand was that the liver is the seat of emotions for the Hmong, not the heart as it is in the West. When the Hmong are heartbroken, it is their livers and stomachs that give them pain.

Cultural differences also affected how nurses cared for Hmong women in labor and delivery. Nurses were perplexed when new Hmong mothers did not urinate after giving birth. Pitchers of ice-cold water were placed on bedside tables but went ignored. When after twenty-four hours the situation had not changed, the doctors became concerned. What they didn't know is that the Hmong believe that hot and cold elements have positive and negative effects on the healing process. In this case, drinking cold water was bad for women who had just given birth. When warm water was served instead, the voiding problem was solved.

Building a small fire under the bed of a new mother or sick person is another Hmong tradition based on the healing properties of heat. On one occasion, a Hmong man pleaded to light a fire under the bed of his seriously ill wife, despite hospital safety regulations. With the help of sympathetic maintenance workers, nurses wheeled the woman in her bed out of the hospital and into an unoccupied area of the attached parking ramp. With the woman's family and a shaman present, the husband lighted the fire. A few minutes later, the ceremony was over, the bed was undamaged, and the family was happy.

Dealing with diseases unheard of in the United States increased stress for physicians who were treating Hmong children. Pediatrician Carolyn McKay, who had worked for two years with the poor in rural Nicaragua, remembers how terrified her St. Paul colleagues were when they had to deal with Hmong children as patients. "They couldn't talk to them," McKay says. "They didn't know what to do about their diseases. They were floored to find that most of the children had worms, often three or more varieties."

McKay remembers receiving a colleague's panicked call one Christmas about a sick child who had just coughed up an *Ascaris,* a worm that looks like a pale angleworm. "If the child is ill and has a fever, the worms try to get out, just like rats leaving sinking ships," explains McKay, who had treated hundreds of children with parasitic worms in Nicaragua. Known locally as the "worm doctor," she began giving lectures on the topic at St. Paul Children's Hospital.

Frustrations with language and cultural differences were growing among the patients too. McKay found that the parents of her Hmong patients were wary of American doctors and the medicine they practiced. "[The Hmong] came out of the seventeenth century, basically," she says of their challenges in adapting to a new culture and a new climate. "At the hospital we had a cupboard that we kept stuffed with used, donated little kids' clothing. I would often unzip a snowsuit and find a naked baby in it when it was twenty degrees below zero outside. People were wearing flip-flops in the snow because they had always dressed that way." Many Hmong women who worked in their yards in the summer did so bare-chested, as they had done back in Laos. Most breast-fed their children beyond infancy, as they had always done.

The Hmong also had a hierarchy in their minds of which medicines and treatments were stronger. When they were sick, they wanted strong medicine, which meant an IV. Next in potency was an injection. Pills were a distant third. The idea that a disease could be chronic was poorly understood. The refugee believed that if he became sick, he could take medicine and then he should not be ill any longer. Why, he wondered, did he have to continue to take medicine when he felt well? Was it because the doctor could not cure him?

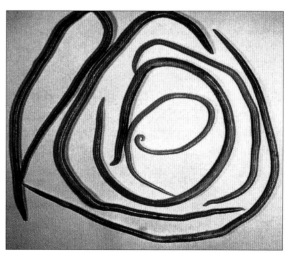

The *Ascaris* worm, a parasite that afflicted many of the refugees in the Thai refugee camps. Pat Walker occasionally saw children pulling the worms out of their noses.

Treating tuberculosis was particularly challenging. The strict regimen requires the infected person to take multiple medications every day for six months or longer, with no gaps in the sequence. If the pills aren't taken as prescribed, the patient can either succumb to the disease or the bacterial organism can become resistant to the drug. Drug-resistant TB can threaten an entire population. The strict regimen is so important from a public-health perspective that many TB patients are required to take their medications under the watchful eye of a nurse. This worldwide standard of treatment is based on a program developed in Singapore called "direct observation therapy." Steve Miles and his colleague, Bob Maat, figured out how to make the DOT program work in an open refugee camp where compliance was supposed to be impossible. Its 98 percent success rate has made it the cornerstone of care not only for refugees with TB, but also HIV and other infectious diseases.

All of this flashed through Neal Holtan's mind when an elderly Hmong patient told Holtan that he was "going to Wisconsin" and couldn't take his TB medicine any longer. Why travel should interfere with taking medications was a mystery to Holtan until another doctor who talked with the man's family learned that "going to Wisconsin" was the Hmong equivalent of "going on the wagon": to stop doing something. The figurative expression had a literal origin: to escape a family problem, a Hmong person from Minnesota might get away to visit relatives who had resettled in Wisconsin. Once Holtan understood the expression, he was better able to explain the hazards of not taking the drug to the man's family, who then agreed to monitor his pill-taking. "If you don't understand the culture, even knowing the language is not going to help," he observes.

Holtan modified the way he conducted himself with his Hmong patients. "One way I worked with my refugee patients was to negotiate: 'If you will do this, then I will do that.' Often I was able to drop things I really did not care about anyway. Let's say a patient needed a medicine and it is customary for everyone who takes that medicine to come back to the clinic every month for a blood test. My patients did not like coming to the clinic and they did not like blood tests. So I would say, 'If you will take this medicine, I will be willing to let you come back every two months and have only a blood test every four months.' By getting down to that kind of level, I found that my patients changed their attitude right there. They felt that they had some kind of control and were not just being ordered to do things. No one wants people controlling them or their children."

But Holtan was the exception. The gulf between cultures and world views was growing. What the hospital needed, Holtan reasoned, was a clinic that would take care of "anyone who has a language or cultural difference that presents a barrier to getting competent medical care."

A Clinic for Immigrants

Holtan brought his clinic idea to Dr. Bob Mulhausen, the same hospital administrator who, just a few months earlier, threatened to fire him when Holtan announced he wanted to join the ARC 15 team. Mulhausen was not only the director of St. Paul–Ramsey Medical Center, he was also its chief of medicine. Not much happened at the hospital that he didn't know about. He was well aware of the growing problems between his staff and their Hmong patients. To Mulhausen, opening a clinic for immigrants made sense. It had as much to do with the bottom line as the Hippocratic oath.

"Bob was very open to us starting the clinic," Holtan remembers. "He wanted it to be not just the medicine department, but to contain both pediatrics and obstetrics—to be cohesive and family-oriented. He also did not want it to be just for Southeast Asians. That was a very smart thing. We did not want the clinic to become a segregated, isolated activity, which was bound to happen if we put each nationality in its own clinic." The International Clinic opened in the fall of 1980, and Mulhausen named Neal Holtan its first director. They thought the clinic would last four or five years at the most.

With its founding, the International Clinic began the ongoing process of justifying its existence. Holtan quickly learned who supported the idea of a clinic for non–English-speaking immigrants and who resisted.

Some hospital workers agreed that refugees and immigrants from cultures different from the Scandinavian/German ethos that had dominated Minnesota from its beginning deserved to be cared for. But that agreement did not translate into a willingness to give up some of *their* space in an already over-crowded building for a clinic for foreigners.

The very concept of "foreigner" carried overtones of bias. Their darker skin and glossy black hair set the Hmong immigrants apart from the pale, blond northerners more commonly seen at the hospital. The idea of caring for the Hmong was fine in the abstract, but when they spoke in an unintelligible language, got lost because they couldn't read the hospital signage, presented medical personnel with unfamiliar symptoms, expressed their own ideas

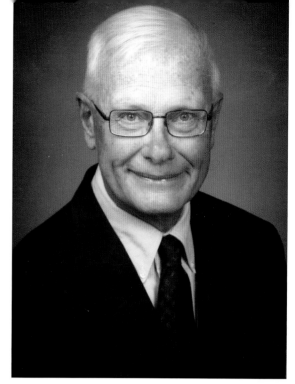

Dr. Bob Mulhausen, director of St. Paul–Ramsey Medical Center.

about what constituted good medical care, and received special attention that had not been provided to other minorities who had been in the country for generations, doctors and nurses backed off or found ways to put up a façade of cooperation.

Holtan remembers that many of the clinic's hurdles were bureaucratic. "A lot of different power centers had to be brought in. Some of them were the nursing administration, the medical staff, the social services department, and the clerical staff. It wasn't as if we had overt resistance. Instead, it was often sort of passive-aggressive: 'Can we really afford this?' they would ask. Or, 'Where is this going to fit into the budget? How much money can be spent on this? You have this employee but only for three-tenths of her time, so who is going to pay for her training?' It was like death by a thousand cuts."

For some objectors, the clinic created more problems than it solved. It added to their workload. It required those who had not had the benefit of a refugee experience to leave the familiar comfort zone of their clinics to work with people elsewhere in the hospital who did not speak English. "Some of the pediatricians could not cope with the fact that their staff was leaving to go to another department to provide care there," Holtan remembers. "They put their objections under the guise of 'not as good quality care.' Nurses maintained that moving the scales from one location to another in the hospital affected the accuracy of the weights, as if that were true or an ounce or two made any difference."

Paramedics also found it difficult to adapt. Back in the early 1980s, the paramedics were an all-male group that was "sort of the macho-cowboy type and they did not want to be bothered with people who did not speak English," Holtan says. "It made their job harder. They had kind of a police mentality. They did not want to deal with people they could not understand and who they could not talk to. They were also resentful when the refugees used them for transportation to the hospital in situations that were not emergencies."

But it was the hospital's surgeons who had the most trouble dealing with culturally different patients. "In personality and style, surgeons are not warm and fuzzy," Holtan observes. "They do their work when people are under anesthesia and it is probably a good thing. They are swashbucklers, action-oriented people who have no time for even gray zones. They did not do well with the refugees in things like getting consent from a family for surgery. The surgeons would try to steamroll them. They would have tantrums, scream at and threaten them."

The pediatricians and psychiatrists were most supportive among his colleagues, Holtan recalls. "Dr. Carolyn McKay, who had a master's of public health from Johns Hopkins, and her boss, Dr. Homer Venters, were wonderful. We had the chief of pediatrics and the chief of medicine supporting us, as well as Laura Edwards, a doctor in obstetrics. We could not have done it without their support." The same was true of the psychiatrists, who treated many Hmong patients for posttraumatic stress disorder and depression.

Piece by piece, maneuvering carefully around the opposition, Neal Holtan put the International Clinic together. But he was still missing the most important component: interpreters. Early on he had decided that the clinic would never use family members as interpreters. There would be no more children translating matters of adult health for their parents. For interpreters Holtan wanted people who could bring more than their language skills to the process. He wanted interpreters who had lived the lives of his patients, interpreters who understood not only the language and the culture but the suffering that had taken place, people who knew how it felt to lose a homeland and have to make their way as strangers in a strange new land. Holtan wanted interpreters who viscerally grasped the immigrants' culture shock—like the young Minnesota man who did not leave his sleeping bag at the refugee camp for three days because he was so overwhelmed by his experience.

Though Holtan did not know it at the time, some of the help he was looking for was already in St. Paul. One such person was Mao Heu Thao, who had arrived in Minnesota four years earlier, pregnant and terrified and not speaking a word of English.

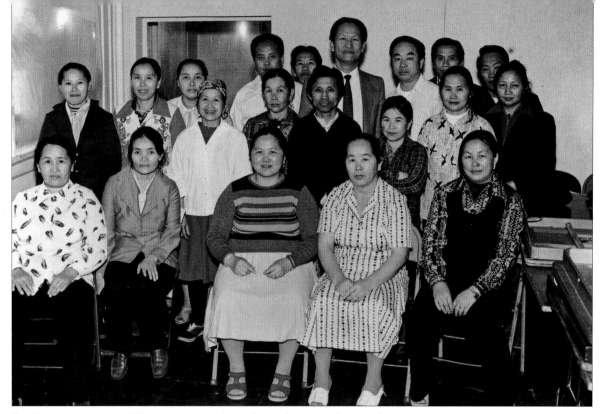

The first graduating class of Hmong women at the Lao Family Community Center in St. Paul, 1981. The center provided classes to help incoming Hmong families adjust to life in Minnesota.

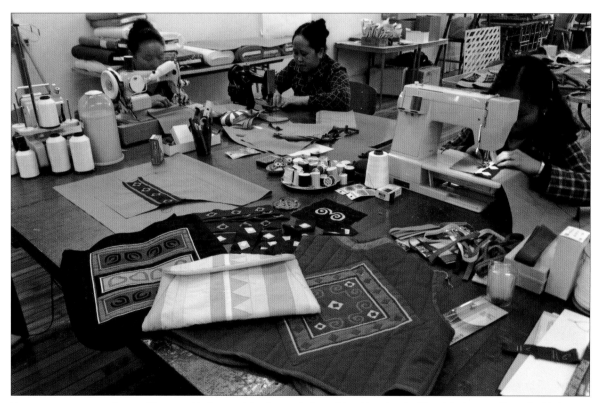

Hmong women use sewing machines to add piecework borders to their traditional hand-embroidered designs, making saleable items such as wall hangings and pillow covers.

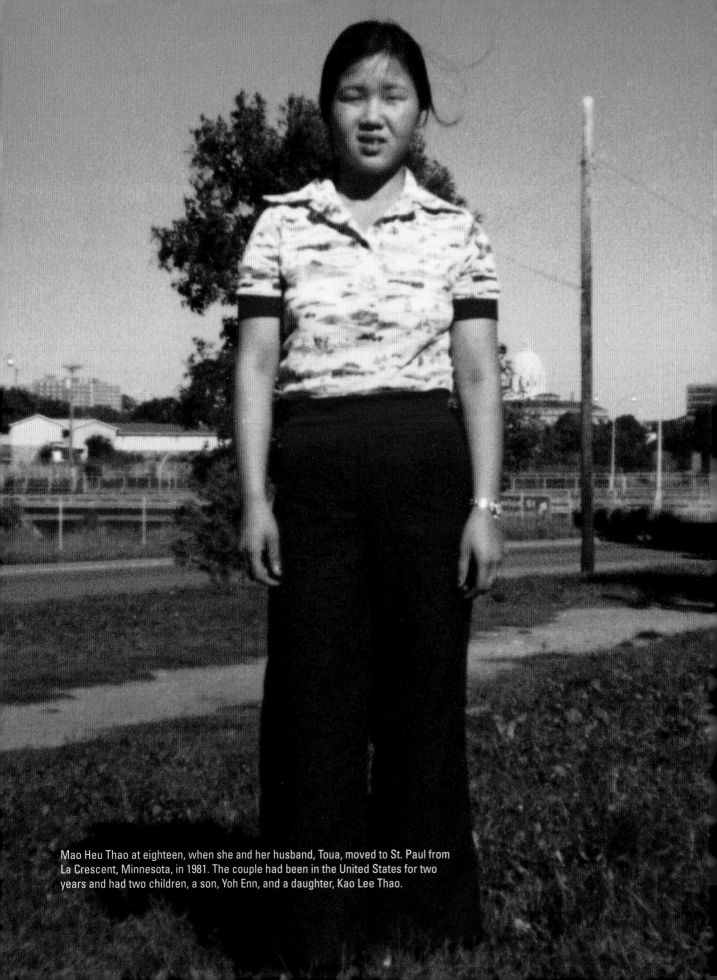

Mao Heu Thao at eighteen, when she and her husband, Toua, moved to St. Paul from La Crescent, Minnesota, in 1981. The couple had been in the United States for two years and had two children, a son, Yoh Enn, and a daughter, Kao Lee Thao.

4: Mao Heu Thao

MAO HEU THAO cannot remember when, as a child, she was not a refugee. Her father, Boua Tong Heu, was a Hmong village chief who fought alongside the Americans in their secret war against the Communists in Laos. As a result, Thao, her parents, and her ten brothers and sisters were constantly on the run, slipping in and out of one village after another, always at night, holding onto each other's hands or shirts as they crept, single-file and silent, through the dark jungle. "We could not use lights of any kind," she remembers, "or we could be caught and killed."

When a village in which they had been living for several months was bombed, all of the residents fled. "My parents left us children in the jungle and crept back to the town to gather more food," Thao says. "They told us not to move. Since we did not want to be killed or separated from our family, we stayed tight together, not moving, all day. Our parents came back to us in the night."

She was married when she was thirteen to Toua Thao, a young man who also worked for the Americans. When the Communists took over Laos after the American withdrawal from Southeast Asia in 1975, the Hmong people were systematically hunted down and killed. Mao's family realized that, to survive, they would have to flee Laos and cross the Mekong River into Thailand. For a price, a Laotian police officer offered to help them and several other families escape to the border.

One morning the officer loaded his human cargo of thirty refugees into the back of a large open truck and struck out for the border. The trip took all day, with frequent stops to push the truck through the mud and to hurry into the jungle when danger threatened. It was nightfall when they reached the river. The officer told the refugees to hide in the jungle and not come out until they heard his signal. Late at night they heard the signal and came running to the riverbank to find boats waiting to take them across the Mekong.

The refugees were about to depart when Mao's husband counted the passengers and discovered that three people were missing: his mother, a three-year-old child, and an infant of four months. The boatmen wanted to leave the three behind rather than risk being discovered by Thai soldiers patrolling the area. Mao's husband leaped ashore to find the missing trio while her brother handed the boatman extra money as further incentive.

After a brief search the three were found and all made it safely across the Mekong River.

They arrived on the Thai bank in the midst of a tropical downpour and took shelter under a chicken coop, where Mao remembers the chicken offal, feathers, and dirt that fell on them with the rain. The next morning they made their way to the Sao Kaeo refugee camp. "There were thousands of people in the camp, some of whom we knew," Mao remembers. "They took us in and gave us shelter. I got malaria and had fever and chills every day." After a few weeks they transferred to the Ban Vinai camp, where Mao and her husband were interviewed for immigration.

"We were ready to leave," she says. "We knew there was no life for us in the camp. There were no jobs. We were surrounded with wire and could not farm or do anything. Because we had been involved with the U.S. government, we were at great risk and could not go back to Laos. The time we were proud that my family had worked for the U.S. government was when we were in the camp and the officials told us, because of what my father and husband had done, we could immigrate. Their names were on a list."

Mao Thao was sixteen years old and seven months' pregnant on March 16, 1976, when she and her husband arrived in the United States. Their sponsor, Catholic Charities of

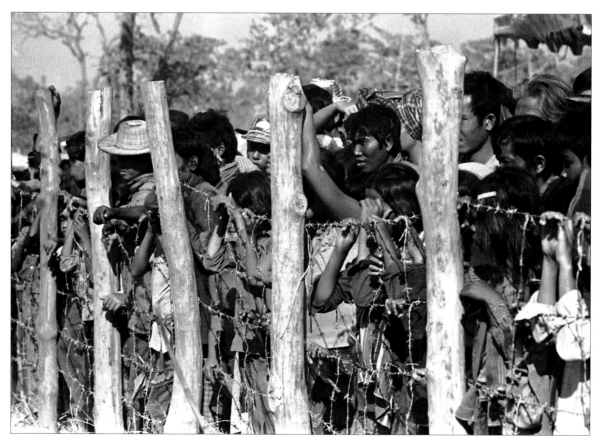

Refugee camps were enclosed with barbed-wire. This photo of Khao I Dang refugee camp is similar to the Ban Vanai camp to which Mao's family fled.

La Crescent, Minnesota, "met us at the airport and drove us to Winona. I was so hungry, but did not know how to ask for food. They took us to a restaurant and asked us what we wanted to eat, but I did not know any words in English to tell them. Also, I was so exhausted from the trip that I could not eat. They took us to a motel for the night and the next day they took us to a couple of churches to look for clothes and shoes. We were both so scared. We did not know what to expect. We did not understand that we could get free clothes and free shoes. The church ladies kept bringing things to us and saying, 'Take them, take them.'"

By 1979, Mao, her husband, and their two children were settled in St. Paul. When Mao learned that Gaoly Yang, the sole Hmong interpreter at St. Paul–Ramsey Medical Center, was leaving for another position, she and her friend, Xiong My Ly, both interviewed for the job and were hired at the same time. Their arrival coincided with the founding of the International Clinic.

Language and Cultural Brokers

When Mao Thao and Xiong My Ly signed on to be interpreters, they assumed they would work forty hours a week. The reality was far different. One hundred thousand Hmong had settled in Minnesota in the last half of 1978, and most of them in the Twin Cities. The International Clinic was swamped. "We worked day in and day out," Thao explains. "We were running all day. The Hmong and Laotian people did not know much about Western culture, so they were afraid of the system, afraid of going to the clinic, afraid of making appointments or seeing a doctor.

"We were on call 24/7. Patients would call us at home if they were to have surgery and ask, 'Should we have the operation? What do you think?' We would explain that we were only interpreters, there to help them communicate with the doctors, relay the messages." Despite the interpreters' disclaimers, anyone who felt sick or in pain would call them. "They didn't call their doctors or their health-care providers," Mao says. "They called their interpreters. Back and forth. It was very stressful.

"One day a two-month-old Hmong baby was brought into the pediatric clinic. The baby had blue Mongolian spots on it, on its arms and at the base of its spine. [Blue spots on the skin are common on Asian newborns.] The young doctors had never seen a baby with Mongolian spots and thought the child was being abused. They called in Child Protection workers and social workers." Thoroughly frightened, the family members tried to protect their child. "They were not used to having to deal with the law, and they were very afraid of doctors and nurses. They did not trust them or the government either, for that matter. The talk about removing the infant from the home was terrible for them. I had to calm the families down, educate the doctors that these blue spots were normal, relay the information back and forth.

"Prenatal care was a huge problem for the Hmong," Thao adds. "We were not used to seeing a doctor when we were pregnant. We believe that nature will take its course and there is no need for a woman to go in every month to see a doctor. Having to get undressed and be examined by a male doctor was a very big deal. Xiong My and I had

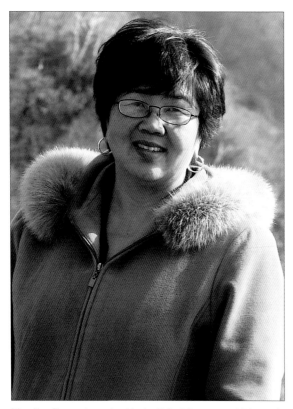

Mao Heu Thao, who arrived in the United States as a frightened, pregnant sixteen-year-old bride, now holds degrees in nursing and health education and program administration. She directs programs for the Hmong community for the St. Paul–Ramsey County Department of Public Health.

to deal with husbands who did not trust their wives and did not trust the doctors. They worried that something bad went on when their wives went to the examining room.

"Using birth control was another big issue," Mao says. "A Hmong wife cannot use birth control without consulting with many people—her husband, her parents, and her in-laws." When the pill was prescribed, it wasn't always used properly. When a young man came into the clinic quite sick and was asked what medicines he was taking, he replied through Mao, "I took some of my wife's medicine." The medicine, he explained, was his wife's birth control pills.

The young man had gone to a Hmong wedding ceremony, a festive occasion celebrated with much alcohol. Someone had told him that if he took birth control pills before taking a drink, he would not get drunk.

Frequently a patient would explain a medical problem to the interpreter, then plead, "But don't tell the doctor!" Mao was interpreting for a man who was supposed to be taking his TB medications. He told the interpreter that he had not taken the medications for a week because he was taking Hmong herbal medicine instead. He added that she was not to inform the doctor. "It is very important for you to take the TB meds, but it is not my job to tell the doctor," Mao told him. "It is OK for you to tell the doctor that you stopped." The man took her advice. "All he needed to hear was that it was OK to tell the doctor that he was taking other medicines—trying to get well."

Clinic interpreters were quick to recognize those doctors who had had overseas experience in refugee camps. "There was much more understanding from these doctors," Mao says. "They would take more time with their patients. Those doctors who knew what the patients had experienced in their lives were different from the others. They would ask questions and sometimes patients would tell them their whole story. Other doctors were impatient, did not have time, and did not want to know anything about their patients. They just wanted a yes or a no.

"Family physicians were more often patient and kind while surgeons were abrupt. Many times a surgeon would say, 'You will die in three days,' or 'You will die in a month or two months.' It was very difficult for us as interpreters to relay that information to a Hmong person because in our culture we don't mention death and dying. People believe that by talking about it, mentioning it, you will bring a curse—make it happen. How do you interpret that to a patient? The Hmong believe only God knows when we will die.

"We would be in a conference room full of Hmong people, the patient's family, and doctors. The patient's family is asked by the doctors to make a decision in a few minutes and the family members say they need many hours. . . .

"In the Hmong community the patient himself cannot make the decision. He has to rely on family members to help. No one wants to be blamed. If the husband decides for the wife and then if something goes wrong after surgery, the woman's family will blame the husband for having given permission for the doctors to perform the procedure. So no one dares to make the decision by himself because if something bad happens, the responsibility for it will be on him.

"The tension between the two groups would be very high. The patient's family would ask, 'What percentage of people survive this surgery? If my wife has this surgery will she survive 100 percent?' Of course, doctors never say surgery is risk-free. They can't promise 100 percent. The Hmong family replies, 'If you cannot say 100 percent, I am not going to allow my wife to have the surgery.' And so the conference would go on for hours and hours. It was exhausting. . . . The interpreters had to be responsive to all the questions and people."

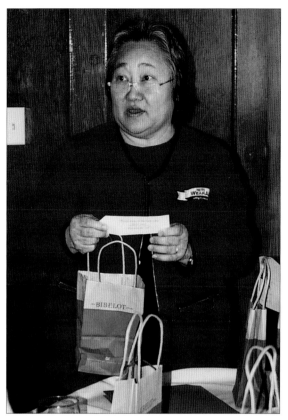

Xiong My Ly at her retirement party in 2006. Xiong was one of the first two Hmong interpreters hired by St. Paul–Ramsey Medical Center in 1979.

"The Hmong were also very opposed to having any metal pieces in the body," Neal Holtan adds. "They cannot be buried in a traditional funeral with metal inside them. That caused a lot of difficulties with plates in heads, pacemakers, artificial hips. We got around it by assuring them that it could all be removed. It helped the situation when we acknowledged that this was a real problem."

Holtan credits the interpreters for the success of the International Clinic. "They were key to the whole thing. They were cultural brokers as well as interpreters and had a calming effect on the patients. They were just what we needed, never interfering, never getting angry with patients. The patients felt that they had someone there who was on their side and understood them. Later it became obvious that the interpreters were indeed neutral, which was hard for the patients to accept at first since they often saw 'sides' between the doctors and their patients.

"The interpreters tried as hard as they could not to pass judgment on anyone. Sometimes they could hardly control themselves when they knew the patient was lying. But they never let that show during the interview."

Emotional Healing

When Neal Holtan founded the International Clinic, he thought he and his staff would be spending most of their time dealing with the physical ailments of immigrants and refugees. As compelling as the organic problems were, the psychological distress was often more acute. As American Refugee Committee volunteer Monica Overkamp discovered when she left Thailand and began working with refugees in the United States, "A lot of them did not experience the symptoms of [posttraumatic stress disorder] until they got here. In the camps they had been living with a lot of stress, coping and surviving and taking care of their families. When they got to the U.S. and found that they were safe, they sort of collapsed. They were not fighting to keep their children alive any more. Those stresses were gone and now other things came to the fore."

Holtan observed that phenomenon as well. "It took us quite a while to figure out what our patients' needs were. We were dealing with problems that other people in the hospital did not see. . . . Families would come

in, desperate for help with a family member who was suicidal, not eating, or becoming violent."

Jim Jaranson, a psychiatrist with a master's in anthropology, first tried meeting with his patients in the psychiatry department, which was housed in a separate building of the hospital. To Jaranson's surprise, the patients failed to show up. "They did not want to be identified as having mental health problems," he explains. "Then I talked with Neal and decided to try seeing the patients in the International Clinic. They could sit in the waiting area just like everyone else and no one knew they were seeing a psychiatrist."

Jaranson became concerned that some mental-health workers may have been trying to force Western therapeutic practice standards upon people who were unfamiliar with them. "I thought we needed to do much more with community-based interventions and self-help programs, get people organized into communities to help them solve some of the problems themselves," he says. "Medication helps. Sometimes counseling does. But I believe group counseling helps much more than individual counseling. Getting together in groups is a concept that many non-Western people are familiar with."

The psychiatrists also worked with shamans, traditional Hmong healers who performed their ceremonies in the patients' rooms. "Unfortunately, that drove some of the nurses and hospital staff crazy," Holtan admits. "The healers brought in food that was not authorized, they burned incense, they drummed. We did draw one line and did not let them sacrifice animals in the hospital."

While Holtan and Jaranson were trying to help their emotionally traumatized patients at the newly formed International Clinic, Minnesota's governor Rudy Perpich, his son Rudy Jr., and an Amnesty International volunteer at Stanford University law school also began talking about what Minnesota could do for refugees. For advice, Governor Perpich contacted the Minnesota Lawyers International Human Rights Committee (now Minnesota Advocates for Human Rights). The group brought in the University of Minnesota law school and its dean, Robert Stein, whose strongest recommendation was to establish the first treatment center for victims of torture in the United States. For advice on how to proceed, Perpich led a delegation to Copenhagen, Denmark, to visit that city's Rehabilitation and Research Center for Torture Victims. Neal Holtan and Jim Jaranson were intimately involved in planning Minnesota's center in 1985.

In the beginning, the Center for Victims of Torture consisted of a Minneapolis office run by Barbara Chester, who held a doctorate in genetic psychology and had experience running a rape crisis center. Local attorneys referred victims to her for evaluation and treatment and she sent most of them on to Holtan and Jaranson at the International Clinic. "When the Center for Victims of Torture started, it did not have a facility where victims could be helped, so the International Clinic at Ramsey took it on," Holtan explains. "We already had torture victims among the refugees we were seeing."

"At first, no one was skilled in treating torture victims," Jaranson says. "Few of us were attuned to the problems of torture survivors until they came to this country. We learned from our patients. We discovered that it is difficult to get information from victims about how they have been tortured. They are very fearful. They will confide in you over time. but first you have to develop a relationship and be patient. They will talk after they feel comfortable with you. . . .

"Most of the Hmong had not been tortured, but the Cambodians were. . . . The whole country was traumatized. Everyone had relatives who were killed. The problems were many and pretty much overwhelming. No single practitioner could attend to all of them." But for a long time Jaranson was the only psychiatrist connected with the Center for Torture.

The two organizations, the Center for Victims of Torture and the International Clinic, worked well together because there was so much overlap between the physical and the psychological problems of their patients. For years internal medicine and psychiatry were the core of the clinic. Jaranson and Holtan saw the torture center's patients at the International Clinic from 1985 until May 1987, when, thanks to a challenge grant from the Northwest Area Foundation and the gift of a house on the University of Minnesota campus, the center opened its own facility. Jaranson and Holtan also took referrals at the hospital after 1987 for specialized medical needs that could not be met at the Center for Victims of Torture house.

"People get better, but they are changed forever. There is an inability to trust other people.

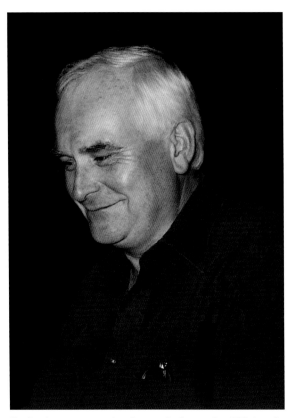

Dr. Jim Jaranson treated patients at the International Clinic and helped found the Center for Victims of Torture in Minneapolis.

One of the big questions in the field is how much of the difficulty refugees have is due to what happened to them before they came and how much is due to all the problems they have adjusting here. Both issues are problems and neither can be ignored."

Growing Pains

Organizationally, it was not always smooth going for the International Clinic. To the hospital administration, the clinic was a messy, expensive undertaking that used resources and occupied space that could be put to better use serving the hospital's more conventional (and intelligible) clientele.

"There have been obstacles over the years because, despite what they say, institutions are not set up to be very interdisciplinary," Jaranson says. "There are always issues on how to work within other departments, who pays for what, and how much you have to bill. Financial constraints grew greater and greater. And there were space issues. At one point the internal medicine department wanted to boot us out because there wasn't enough space. The International Clinic was part of internal medicine, but I was part of psychiatry. We talked them out of closing us down."

To the refugees and immigrants, the clinic was a lifeline and a portal into the puzzling new world of the United States. Every year, more and more of them came to the International Clinic. In 1987 more than two thousand immigrants came through the clinic doors, bringing with them not only their medical complaints, but all of the bureaucratic problems that attended their legal status in the United States.

Holtan found dealing with citizenship issues "just horrible." Even adults needed letters from their doctors documenting immunizations and explaining their absence from English classes. The state required immigrants receiving financial assistance either to enroll in an English language class or to hold a job. (It was especially difficult for Asian women to understand why they could be forced to take a job in a factory or a fast-food chain when what they wanted was to take care of their children and households.) Waivers excusing an adult from having to gain proficiency in English as a prerequisite for citizenship had been established to deal with such situations as an elderly grandmother who, despite her best efforts, could not remember a word of English. However, for the waiver to be approved, doctors had to first determine if there were medical conditions that prevented the woman from learning English.

"I spent a fourth of my time signing forms for the county, certifying disability and things like that," Holtan laments. He and other doctors spent hours filling out multi-page forms, dictating a patient's entire medical history and stating the medical reason that they could not learn English. Patients brought their forms with them into the examining rooms and would not leave until the doctors dealt with them.

While there were many complex aspects to dealing with the welfare system on behalf of his patients, the issue that came the closest to driving Holtan crazy was public housing. "The housing authorities have very strict and unbending rules and bureaucrats who enforce them," he says. "They are inundated with people who have special requests. 'I want a bigger apartment' or 'I can't sleep in this room.' Whenever the bureaucrats got totally frustrated they would say, 'Well, get a letter from your doctor.' We were dumped on as the last resort whenever our patients were frustrated with welfare or the housing authorities."

Holtan's most frustrating experience during his early years at the clinic involved one of his patients, a veteran of the South Vietnam army whose legs had been blown off by a bomb. He also had suffered severe damage to his arms, so in effect he had neither functioning arms nor legs. Holtan wanted to get the man a motorized wheelchair

because his family were not able to push him up the ramp to their house in a non-motorized chair. Holtan began calling and writing letters. Months passed and authorization for the wheelchair never came. Finally, he called the Minnesota commissioner of human services and said, "You *have* to do something about this." She did, and the man finally got his wheelchair.

"This is a lot of what we did in the International Clinic," Holtan explains. "It was not so much medicine as taking care of these other things. This is why all those inefficiencies occurred in our clinic. The staff in those clinics were there only for disease-oriented issues. We dealt with *everything.*"

By the end of 1987, the International Clinic had served thousands of patients. Although some physicians still opposed Holtan's project, he found that others were happy to refer their patients to him and his staff. These physicians knew that they could get information and support from the clinic staff about diseases they rarely saw in the United States. Although some doctors still scratched their heads when a patient spoke in her own language for three minutes only to have a translator say, "She says no," many health-care workers trusted the interpreters and worked well with them.

Seven years after founding the International Clinic, Neal Holtan remembered the third-year student who had interrupted her medical education to go to Thailand with the ARC 15. He had been impressed with her compassion and commitment and decided the time had come for him to get back in touch with Pat Walker.

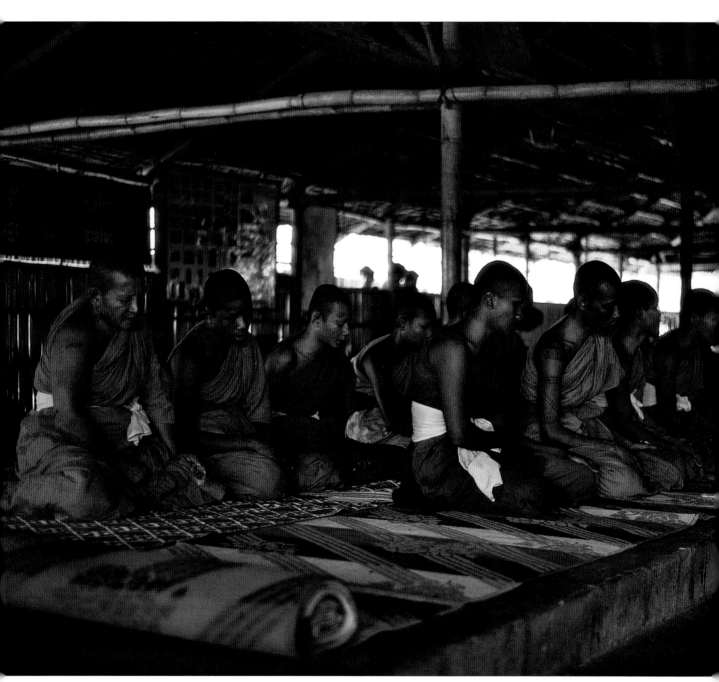

Cambodian monks at the Khao I Dang refugee camp performing a traditional funeral rite of prayers and chanting for a fellow monk, a patient of Pat Walker's, who had died. Before the service the monks had washed and clothed the body and placed it in a wooden coffin so family and friends could pay their respects. Following the ceremony the coffin was placed in the back of a truck and driven in a slow procession to the site of the funeral pyre. Pat Walker and others watched as the pyre was lit and black smoke billowed from the coffin.

5: a year of living dangerously

THOUGH SHE WAS HAPPILY immersed in her education back in Minnesota at Mayo Medical School and was taking advantage of its enormous resources, Pat Walker often wondered what the money spent there could have purchased back at the Khao I Dang refugee camp. She was doing bone marrow biopsies on a special tilt table one day when she realized that the table cost more than the entire hospital she and the rest of the ARC 15 had built for the refugees. Walker determined that when she had completed medical school and paid off her debts, she would return to Southeast Asia and work with refugees.

But if she were to be useful overseas later, Walker realized, she would need broader exposure now to the day-to-day ills of humankind. So while completing the first two years of her residency at Mayo, she moonlighted in the emergency room of a Wisconsin hospital. Early every fourth Saturday morning, Walker drove 110 miles from Rochester to St. Croix Falls for a weekend shift at St. Croix Regional Medical Center. She was on duty thirty-four hours, from noon on Saturday until ten o'clock on Sunday night. Since she was the only physician staffing the emergency room, she was often awake the entire time she was on

duty. Late Sunday night she would drive back to Rochester, arriving at 2:00 a.m.— just four hours before she started work again at the Mayo Clinic.

"I did the ER work for two reasons," Walker explains. "I needed the money—I had put myself through medical school— and I wanted to be a good generalist as well as a good internist. I wanted to be able to look in kids' ears and sew up a wound and diagnose appendicitis."

When she finished her internal medicine residency at Mayo in 1984, Walker worked as an emergency room doctor in Mason City, Iowa, and then became medical director of the ER at Mount Sinai Hospital in Minneapolis. After three years at Mount Sinai, she felt that she was ready to return to Thailand.

When Neal Holtan told Walker that he wanted her to work with him at the International Clinic, she was torn. She had a burning desire to get back to Thailand, but knew that she would probably not want to stay there forever. She agreed to an interview with Dr. Kent Crossley, chief of internal medicine at St. Paul–Ramsey Medical Center, and found him to be "an outstanding physician who really understood that the global is local in health care." At the end of the interview, she agreed to return to St. Paul after a year in Thailand and work with Holtan in the clinic.

Outpatient Department 7

By October 1987, Pat Walker was back in Khao I Dang, this time as medical director for the International Rescue Committee, the same organization that years earlier had helped Neal Ball, ARC's founder, visit Thailand to find members of Phunguene Sananikone's family.

"The IRC is a wonderful organization, formed in the 1930s to help Jews escaping from Germany," Walker says. "It is the leading nonsectarian medical organization around the world, and it is huge." She directed a

staff of thirty-five Cambodian medical assistants, most of whom had been trained in the education program that Steve Miles and his colleagues established during their American Refugee Committee tour.

Returning to Thailand was like going home for Walker. Her older sister, Susan Walker, who had dropped everything in 1979 to become the overseas director for the American Refugee Committee, was still there, now serving as chair of the coordinating committee for all NGOs (fifty-two at its peak) that worked with displaced people in Thailand. Meanwhile, Pat and Susan's younger sister, Elizabeth Walker Anderson, was working for the International Rescue Committee. Elizabeth's husband, Jim Anderson, was the IRC country chair for Thailand and Pat's boss.

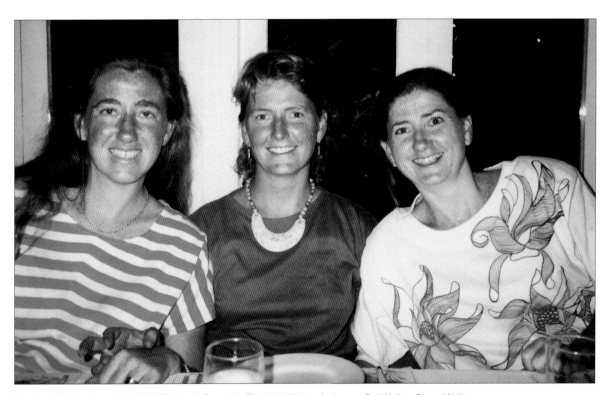

The three Walker sisters in 1988 in Thailand. From left: Elizabeth Walker Anderson, Pat Walker, Susan Walker.

"my heart it is delicious"

"Jim, Liz, and Susan all shared a house in Bangkok, so when I went back to Thailand in 1987, I had a home to go to and family to be with," Pat Walker says. At the time, she was the highest paid physician working for the International Rescue Committee. She earned $1,250 a month, $1,000 of which she sent home to pay off her debts.

She worked in Khao I Dang camp's Outpatient Department 7, a large, L-shaped bamboo building covered with a thatched roof. Patients began lining up before dawn. By 7:30 hundreds of refugees would be waiting to enter through a small triage area where Cambodian medics diagnosed and treated patients on the spot. When the medics encountered complicated cases, they brought them to Walker or to one of the other two American physicians in the camp.

"We probably had four hundred patients a day," Walker remembers. "Each medic would see about forty patients a day, and out of every ten they saw they would send one or two of the sickest to me. I stood at the juncture of the L and examined patients right there, out in the open. There were forty people watching me all of the time. There was no privacy."

It was here, in the very public juncture of the L, that a monk with severe abdominal pain was brought to Walker. "Now what do I do?" she wondered. She knew she wasn't supposed to touch a Buddhist monk. Monks considered women to be unclean and had to undergo a special ceremony to cleanse themselves if touched by a woman. Fortunately for Walker, there were a few private examining areas along the back wall of the clinic. Accompanied by several men as wit-

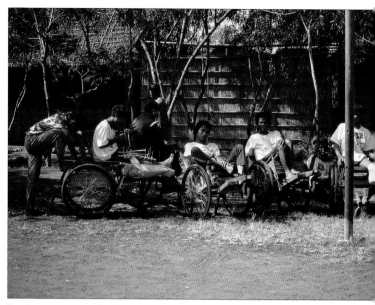

One in twenty-seven Cambodians lost limbs to land mines. Above: amputees at Khao I Dang in handmade wheelchairs. Below: a three-legged race in camp.

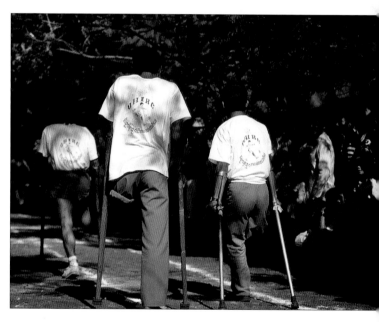

nesses, she took the monk into a small room, where he agreed to her examination. When she finished, she apologized to him for having to touch his abdomen. She diagnosed a probable ulcer, but never learned if he went through with a cleansing ceremony after her exam.

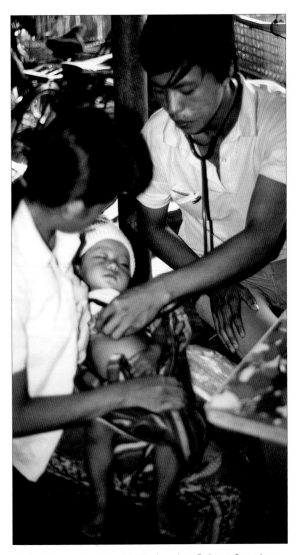

Cambodian medics, trained in the American Refugee Committee classes, attend patients at Khao I Dang camp.

An aura of thinly veiled anxiety, of hope bordering on desperation to attract the attention of an American sponsor, engulfed the medics. With elaborate casualness they would quiz each new American arrival. "Where are you from? Do you have children? Do you have a big house?" The refugees' pointed questions prompted long philosophical discussions between Pat and Susan Walker that raised questions of their own: How could individual Americans best provide help for the displaced? What is one person's responsibility? Was it better to work at the big picture of helping many refugees or to help a single individual?

As Pat Walker considered her own situation (she *did* have a big house in Minneapolis), she decided she would help one of the Cambodian medics who joined her in her work. She was drawn to Monorom Sok Hang, whose intelligence and optimistic spirit had impressed her. Monorom came to work at Department 7 every day by himself, and during their many conversations, Walker got the impression that Monorom was alone in the world. "The real difference about Monorom was that he did not have a family," she recalls. "That got to me."

Walker was impressed with the medics working in Outpatient Department 7. "These were a group of smart, energetic, young people, the most successful people in the camp. They had gotten training to learn how to do a prestigious job, were eager to learn more, and were receiving extra food and a small amount of pay for their work. They were all about twenty years old, and every single one of them was absolutely focused on the goal of going to the United States."

Following long discussions with her own family, Walker decided that, when she returned to the United States, she would sponsor Mono, as he was called, and bring him home to live with her. She told herself that she was good at setting boundaries; that she would not become a parent to Mono, who was already an adult, but that she would commit to helping him find a job and learning about life in America. Completing the paperwork for him to immigrate would be easy since her sister Elizabeth was running the

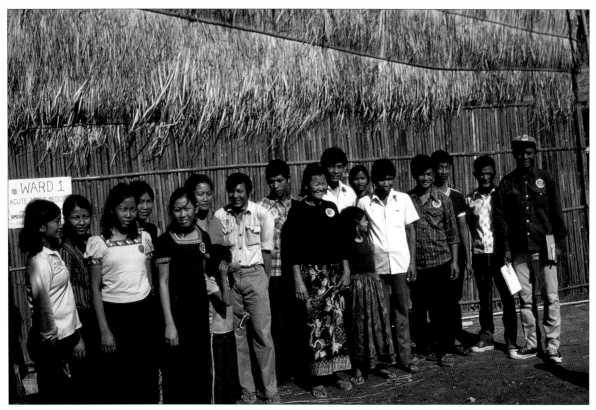

The staff of ARC refugee medical workers outside a thatch-walled hospital building at Khao I Dang.

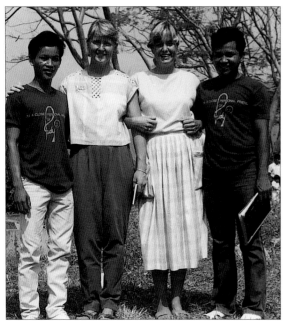

Dr. Pat Walker and program coordinator Monica Overkamp with graduating medics Monorom Sok Hang and Yan Yunn.

Cambodian Resettlement Program. One day Pat Walker broke the news to Mono that, if he wished, she would sponsor him. "I will help you," she promised him. Meanwhile, she had work to do in the camp.

Life-or-Death Decisions

In addition to treating the various diseases common in the camp, Walker was on a committee of physicians and nurses whose agonizing task it was to decide which patients would benefit the most from being transferred to another country for treatment via the "Medically at Risk" program. Norway, Sweden, Denmark, Canada, and the United States all had agreed to accept such patients.

Walker looked at her ward of young patients with rheumatic heart disease. Listening to their hearts she heard, over and over again, the distinctive rumbling murmur of mitral stenosis, a narrowing or blockage of the mitral valve. Rheumatic fever and strep infection were the common causes of mitral stenosis. At some time in the past these youth had been sick but had not taken penicillin for the required ten days. Their only option had been to buy their penicillin on the black market. They stopped taking the expensive drug when they felt better, and the untreated infection then damaged their hearts. If they could get new heart valves in open-heart surgery, they could expect to live long, productive lives. Without the surgery, they would be dead in several years.

But another patient had attracted Walker's attention, a tiny Cambodian woman named Veera Som, who was gravely ill with asthma. Veera and her younger sister Channy were well known to the American medical staff who worked at the Ban Nong Samet camp on the Cambodian border and who traveled back and forth between Ban Nong and Khao I Dang. Despite her asthma, Veera had taken the ARC course for medics offered at Ban Nong Samet and had worked in the hospital there for seven years.

When, one day, the American staff spotted Veera and Channy among the refugees in the Khao I Dang camp, they immediately figured out what must have happened. The Thai government had long ago closed Khao I Dang to additional Cambodian refugees. The only way the two sisters could have gotten into Khao I Dang was to have been smuggled in from Ban Nong Samet. They were "illegals," displaced persons rather than refugees, and if caught by the Thai guards they would be punished and forcibly deported to Cambodia. As illegals, Veera and Channy had no legitimate way to get food or be assigned a place to live. They were on their own. Despite the fact the American medical workers were caring for as many as four hundred patients a day, they resolved to keep a watchful eye on Veera and Channy.

"Because there was so much dust, especially in the dry season, asthma in that setting was terrible," Walker remembers. "The only medication we had for asthma was albuterol, an inhaler, and theophylline, a medication Western physicians did not like using because of its side effects. Veera had such bad asthma that she would cough and then have bronchial spasms that could kill her very quickly." Despite living with a constant fear of death and memories of the terrible events she had experienced during the war, Veera was full of energy. "She had bright eyes, a bright smile, and was happy and optimistic," Walker recalls. "My impression was that this was someone who was special. I saw so many people, hundreds a day, but some stood out because they had an energy about them—the energy of a survivor. Somehow, no matter what has happened to them, these people maintain a sense of joy. Veera was like that."

When Walker thought about which patients the committee should choose to transport to another country for medical care, her thoughts always returned to Veera. Before she could do anything about the young woman's case, however, Walker had another, more dangerous situation to resolve.

Smuggling Medical Supplies

In 1987 Vietnam's government allowed hundreds of political prisoners to leave Vietnamese jails, but refused them permission to leave the country. These former prisoners and their families wanted only to get out of Vietnam, and they were prepared to take enormous risks to do so. To the east and south of Vietnam was the South China Sea; to the west was Laos and Cambodia, now occupied by the North Vietnamese. To the north was China. The only avenue of escape was by boat from the south, then west around the southern end of Cambodia to Thailand, where the refugees hoped to find asylum.

This route had been used before, in 1979, when one million "boat people" fled Vietnam. As many as 600,000 were kidnapped, raped, and/or murdered by pirates. Some boatmen were outright bandits; others were poor fishermen whose single teeming boatload of passengers could be worth thousands of dollars. The fisherman knew that the refugees had transferred all of their assets into gold before leaving Vietnam. Once they had their passengers onboard, they robbed them and threw them overboard. Other victims died of starvation, dehydration, and illness. One country, Malaysia, refused to let the refugee-laden boats land, fired cannon at them, and towed the ramshackle crafts back out to sea. At least half of the people who left Vietnam by boat in the late 1970s perished at sea.

Despite the horrific experiences of the first boat people, episodes that shocked the world, the political prisoners who were released in 1987 were undeterred. Knowing that barely half of them were likely to survive the trip, they began escaping Vietnam by sailing to Thailand on any fishing boat that would take them. "We will take you to Thailand," promised the boatmen. What they did not tell their passengers was that they planned to abandon them on Thailand's off-shore islands. Since Thailand had closed its borders to refugees and it was illegal to bring them into the country, the boatmen would sail their watercraft close to the off-shore islands and tell their passengers, "The engines on the boat have died. Jump in and swim to shore."

Jim Anderson, Pat Walker's brother-in-law and the Thailand country director for the International Rescue Committee, had heard rumors that a huge wave of Vietnamese refugees was being landed on the islands. So had Lionel Rosenblatt and John Crowley, staff members at the U.S. Embassy. The Thai government, suffering from what the three men charitably refer to as "compassion fatigue," maintained that nothing at all was going on. The trio decided to find out for themselves what was happening.

They drove to the southern Thai port city of Trat, where they took a boat to visit the string of islands just off Thailand's shore. They stopped first at the largest island, Koh Chang, then visited Ko Samae San, Ko Kut, and Ko Man, interviewing the village chiefs to find out how many Vietnamese refugees were living there, what food supplies they had, and whether many were sick. They learned that Thai fishermen were charging $1,000 a person to bring refugees into Thai waters. The three men found hundreds of Vietnamese, many of them ill, stranded on the islands.

When Anderson returned to Khao I Dang, he told Pat Walker that they had to do something to get medical supplies to the Vietnamese refugees. He asked her if she would be willing to go to the islands, assess the status of the refugees' health, and bring a load of supplies. "If you get caught by Thai officials," he warned, "you'll be kicked out of the country and the International Rescue Committee will probably be thrown out too." Despite the hazards, she agreed to make the trip.

Anderson filled the back of a Toyota truck with medical supplies and covered it with a tarp. To help disguise herself, Walker wore "a big, ridiculous-looking straw hat and big sunglasses" and began the four-hour drive to Trat through the beautiful fruit-plantation countryside of Thailand. The road was dotted with military checkpoints. At each one Walker greeted the guards with a giddy monologue about how she was going to the beach for a weekend with friends. "They never looked in the back of the truck," she says. "I think it was because I was a woman and I acted silly."

Once at the Trat docks, Walker met Anderson, who introduced her to the two Thai men who would accompany her on her visits to the islands. "These nonmedical men were to be my liaisons with the villages," she says. "The chiefs would not let me in to do anything without these men coming with me. They were risking their careers to accompany me." She and her companions began transferring the truck's contents onto a big charter fishing boat, including case after case of bottled water. The sight of the lone American woman and the two Thai men working on the dock attracted atten-

tion, and onlookers began to ask pointed questions. One of the Thai men acted quickly. He pulled one of the questioners aside and explained, sotto voce, "You know, she is one of those strange Americans. She is not going to drink all that water. That is for her showers."

Systematically, Walker and her guides visited each island, lush tropical outposts ringed with white sand beaches and covered with plantations of bamboo and coconut palms. Walker and her companions visited each of the small Thai fishing villages and its chief. The chiefs' responses ran the gamut. Some told her, "I'm a Buddhist and I must help. So I have brought these people in and we are sharing our food and water and shelter with them as best we can." Another village leader said, "I know what to do with these refugees. We should take them all out in the ocean, push them off the boat, and let the sharks take care of them."

It was just after dark when the trio hitched their boat at a dock on one small island where, up a hillside, stood a solitary house built on stilts. The two-room building had thatched walls and a thatched roof. Told by the village elders that Vietnamese refugees were sheltered in the house, Walker and her companions trudged up the hill, climbed the ladder to the entrance, and pushed through the door. Their flashlights revealed seventy-two refugees, staring back at them with apprehension. Some were lying down, others sat shoulder to shoulder, and it was obvious that many were ill. Walker quickly explained to her two helpers that she needed them to take temperatures and pulse rates so she could identify those who needed immediate medical attention. When the men looked dubious—this was not what they had signed on for—she assured them, "You can do this." With their help, she quickly found the fourteen sickest people. They had temperatures of 105 and were probably suffering from malaria.

Walker began hanging bottles of intravenous quinine to treat the malaria patients and IV fluids for those who looked to be dying from dehydration. She instructed the two men to monitor the IVs and to hand out malaria pills to those who probably had the disease but were well enough not to need IV treatment. Sometime after midnight one of the IV patients, a pregnant woman with a temperature of 104 and probable malaria, began to deliver her baby.

Although the woman was full term, the labor was a difficult one and the birthing process tore her vagina. Walker had nothing with her to suture the laceration, so she applied pressure to stop the bleeding. When she realized that she was failing to take care of the other refugees who were critically ill, Walker asked a woman sitting next to her to keep pressure on the tear while she tended other patients. Walker clung to the hope that the woman would stop bleeding and that Walker could evacuate her and her baby in the boat the next morning.

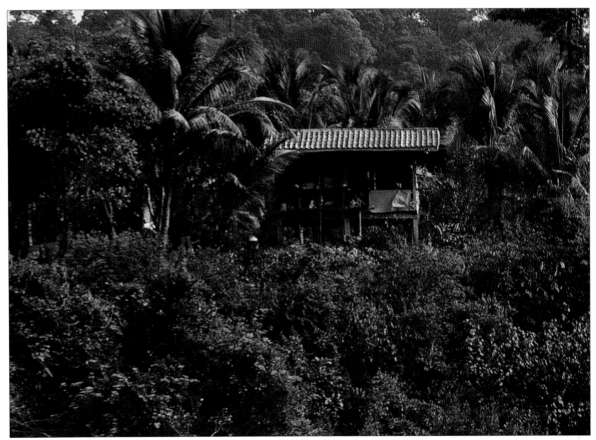

The hut where Dr. Walker discovered seventy Vietnamese refugees taking shelter for the night.

But the woman's condition worsened. "It could have been the malaria, it could have been the quinine," Walker says. "There may have been a drop in her blood sugar, which sometimes can happen with malaria and IV quinine or because her blood count was already low. She was anemic from her malaria and probably anemic from hookworm and she went into a coma." The woman delivered a stillborn girl. Walker tried to resuscitate the baby but without success.

"The baby died, the mom died, and this woman's five-year-old son sat there and watched the whole thing happen," Walker says. "It was just terrible. Two needless deaths! About four in the morning I walked down to the dock. There was a big water jar, and I took a bucket which you use to wash yourself and poured the water over my head and washed off all the blood and meconium that was on me and just sobbed." It remains the most difficult night of her medical career.

The Thai government eventually acknowledged the presence of the Vietnamese refugees on the islands and removed them to the Thai mainland, where they received medical care at the Khao I Dang hospital. It was months before Walker would learn that the father of the boy who had witnessed the deaths of his mother and infant sister had been located and the two reunited.

Going Home
Walker's year in Thailand ended in the summer of 1988. She didn't want to leave, but she had given her word and made her commitment to report to the International Clinic

in August. The person who was the most anxious about her return to Minnesota was Monorom, the Cambodian medic she had agreed to sponsor. "I think my departure scared him to death," she says. "So many Americans in those situations say they will help someone and then they return home and disappear." Though she continually reassured Mono that as soon as she returned to the States she would begin the process to sponsor him, he remained troubled.

Walker learned why Mono was anxious about a week before she left for the United States. In the midst of a busy day at the Khao I Dang outpatient clinic, he came up to her and said, "I have a brother."

She was stunned. She had worked with Mono for a year, yet he had never said anything about his brother. The next day Mono brought Mony to the clinic to meet Walker. Mony was only a year younger than Mono. For a time Walker reconsidered the situation. Were the stories Mono had told her about his past real? What else didn't she know about him? Then she made her decision. "It was understandable that Monorom did not trust that I would sponsor him when I learned he had a relative," she reasoned. "But once he told me, I still trusted him." With the stories of Mono and his brother Mony and of Veera and her sister Channy tugging at her heart, Walker returned to Minnesota.

Another shock awaited her when she reported for work at St. Paul–Ramsey Medical Center and her boss, Neal Holtan, announced, "I'm ready to move on, and I want you to take over the International Clinic. You're now the medical director."

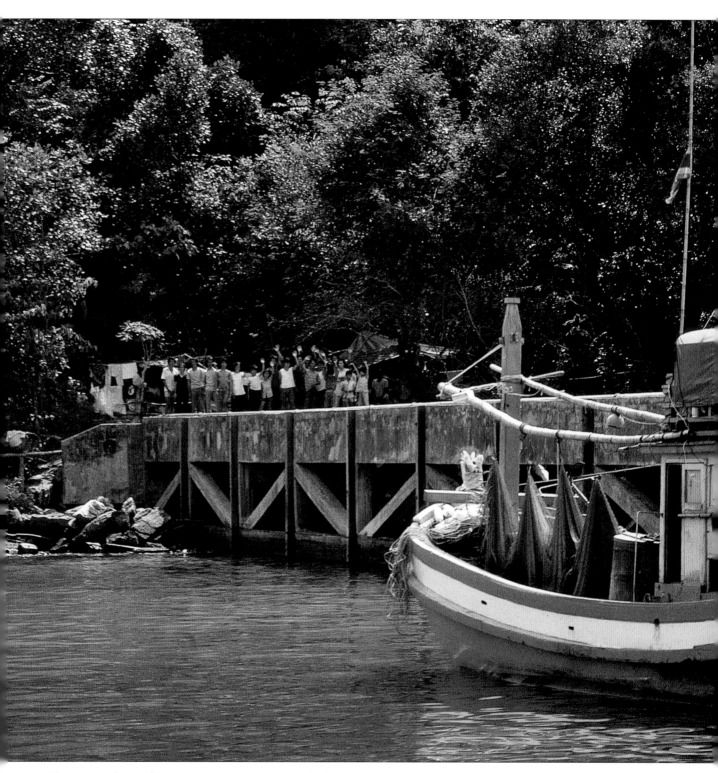

Vietnamese refugees sharing a communal meal on an outlying Thai island wave to Pat Walker as she travels from island to island checking on the refugees' welfare.

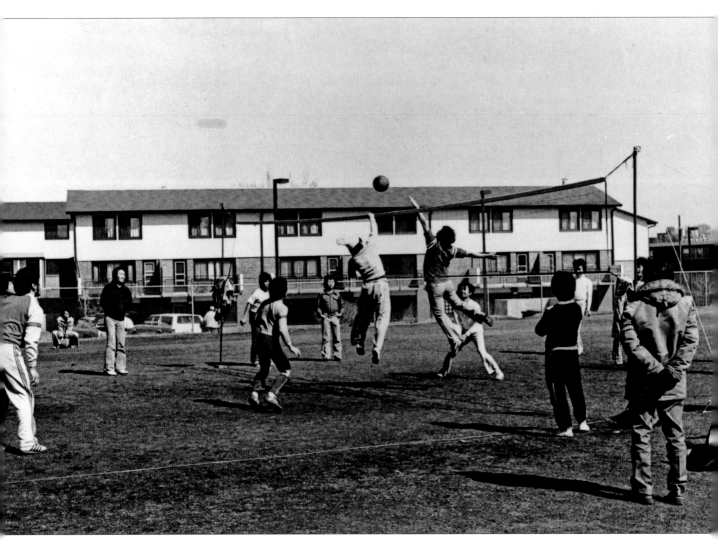

Hmong young people play volleyball at a playground within walking distance of the International Clinic in downtown St. Paul, early 1980s.

6: new directions

PAT WALKER COULD not have been more surprised at Neal Holtan's news that he was stepping down as the medical director of St. Paul–Ramsey's International Clinic. "I walked in thinking I was going to learn from my mentor and instead he put me in charge," she says. Holtan assured her that he would continue seeing patients at the clinic; he just didn't want to deal with the administrative part of the job any longer.

At that time, in August 1988, the clinic was seeing approximately two thousand patients a year. The staff consisted of Holtan and a part-time physician, plus psychiatrist Jim Jaranson and four interpreters: one speaking Hmong and the others speaking Vietnamese, Cambodian, and Spanish. The staff worked Monday through Friday from 8:00 to 5:00. On Tuesday and Thursday, a pediatrician and two pediatric nurse practitioners saw patients from 5:00 until 8:00. The clinic was on the second floor of the medical center, which was no longer a county hospital but a private, not-for-profit facility. The building, much added to over the years, loomed over Interstate 94 at Jackson and University Avenues, an impressive and somewhat forbidding multistoried monument to modern medical care.

Patients waiting to be seen in the International Clinic sat in chairs in the hospital corridor. There was little else to indicate that this hallway was a reception area. No tables were piled with outdated issues of *Reader's Digest* or *People* magazine; no television droned in the background. In front of the waiting patients was a children's play area, walled off from the corridor by an empty counter. On the wall above the play area was a framed Hmong tapestry, a poster welcoming patients in Spanish, Hmong, Cambodian, and Vietnamese, and a framed Patient's Bill of Rights, the latter in English.

Two doors off the corridor led onto two short hallways, each with six examining rooms, three to a side. At the end of the hallways and running parallel to the waiting area was another corridor that served as the doctors' makeshift office. Here, when they were not seeing patients, Pat Walker, Neal Holtan, and Jim Jaranson sat in a row at a cafeteria-style table, writing prescriptions, jotting notes in charts, and completing forms. "People had to squeeze past us to get by in the hall," Walker remembers.

Although the clinic was already well known in the immigrant community, the patient load increased dramatically with Walker's arrival. The refugee grapevine quickly spread the word that a new doctor who spoke "our" language was in town. "The pent-up demand was already there," she observes. "Every time the clinic added capacity, more patients came."

Walker found the work in the clinic both easy and familiar. With 80 to 90 percent of the clinic's patients coming from Southeast Asia, their complaints were remarkably similar to those she had seen in the Khao I Dang camp. Yet she was surprised to find her refugee patients to be basically healthy when compared to Americans. While the immigrants had medical problems related to malnutrition and infectious disease, their underlying physical ailments were unlike the illnesses that plagued most Americans. Doctors call it the "healthy migrant effect": In other words, says Walker, "it takes about nine years for an immigrant to become 'American' in his body—obese, hypertensive, diabetic, and at risk for strokes and heart attacks."

Right Diagnosis, Wrong Treatment

Most patients coming to the International Clinic for the first time were infected with worms, so Walker made sure everyone was tested for parasites. Patients also were tested for tuberculosis, hepatitis B, syphilis, and HIV.

The parasitic worms, mostly roundworms, gave their hosts iron-deficiency anemia as they sucked blood from their intestines. If they were really large worms, they moved into the bile or pancreatic ducts and caused what looked like gallstones or pancreatitis.

Walker was philosophical about the worms. "In the greater scheme of things," she says, "typically those worms will die, and if the patient is living in the U.S., he won't become reinfected." But not all of the worms were benign. There *was* a worm that was extremely dangerous, and if Western doctors did not recognize the symptoms, they could unknowingly kill the patients they were trying to cure.

The worm, called *Strongyloides,* has both male and female larvae and can survive in the human body for more than sixty years. Doctors at the London School of Tropical Medicine discovered the worm in the 1980s and 1990s while treating soldiers who had fought in World War II on the Thai-Burmese railway—the setting for *The Bridge on the River Kwai*. These soldiers experienced a red raised welt across their chests and abdomens that moved in a line; the welt lasted a couple of hours and then went away. It would come back six months or even two years later. The moving line was the worm.

The biggest problem with the *Strongyloides* worm is that it is opportunistic. If the larvae breaks through the intestines, it can migrate to the liver, lungs, and nervous system. As the infection works its way into the bloodstream and spinal fluid, it brings with it bacteria from the gut. The patient gets meningitis or sepsis, a blood infection, and dies. The process of infection is accelerated when the infected person's immune system is compromised, particularly when given steroids for underlying conditions such as emphysema, for which IV steroids are the standard treatment. Over the course of a decade, St. Paul had 160 cases of *Strongyloides.* In five of the cases, physicians treated their patients with IV steroids for emphysema. Three men died before Walker figured out what was happening and could publish her findings in the medical literature.

Through working with patients infected with *Strongyloides,* Walker learned about another peculiarity: patients with the worm have a high count of a particular white blood cell called an eosinophil. If an American has a high eosinophil count, it is an indication he has not worms but asthma. If an Asian has a high eosinophil count, it means he is probably infected with this deadly worm or other worms.

One day, Walker sent a Cambodian patient with an elevated eosinophil count and the *Strongyloides* infection to a hematologist at the hospital for advice on what to do for the patient's complex anemia. The blood specialist wrote back with treatment advice for the anemia and then added, "The patient has a mild eosinophilia—*but I would ignore that.*" Walker's colleague had no idea that, 95 percent of the time, a finding of eosinophilia in an Asian means that the patient has a life-threatening pathogenic parasite. Walker alerted the other staff and resident physicians to the danger. "We had to," she says. "There were more and more immigrants coming, and doctors had to understand and recognize this phenomenon."

Cultural Differences

There was daily conflict and misunderstanding at the International Clinic as Western-trained surgeons, gynecologists, and emergency medicine physicians tumbled into the gulf of cultural differences that separated them from their foreign-born patients.

Walker had been working in the clinic for a few months when she received a phone call from a frustrated surgeon. "Come up

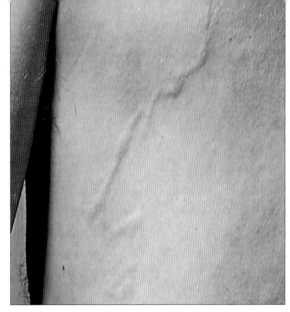

The red welt moving just below the skin is characteristic of the *Strongyloides* worm's presence within the body.

here right away," he angrily demanded. "We have a woman with an ectopic pregnancy and she is refusing surgery." An ectopic pregnancy is one in which the fertilized egg has implanted outside the uterus, usually in the Fallopian tube. Trailed by a Hmong interpreter, Walker went to talk with the woman.

The surgeon had explained to the patient that he would have to take out one of her Fallopian tubes and one ovary with the possibility that the surgery would leave her infertile. If he found additional problems in her abdomen, he would have to remove both ovaries. Without the surgery she would probably die.

"I cannot do that," the woman replied. "I cannot risk being infertile." When Walker asked her why, the woman explained that, although she already had five children, her husband wanted her to have more. In traditional Hmong culture, if the wife is infertile, the husband can divorce her. Furthermore, the children are the property of the father. The woman's choice was, literally, between her husband and children or her life. The woman chose to go home. Remarkably, the pregnancy growing in her tube reabsorbed and she survived, much to Walker's and the surgeon's surprise.

Not every situation had such a fortunate ending. In the 1980s something puzzling began happening to apparently healthy young Hmong men in Minnesota. They would be asleep in their homes when they would suddenly sit up, cry out as if having a nightmare, and then drop dead. Before long, Minnesota had 150 cases of what was called sudden unexplained death syndrome, or SUDS. Autopsies (mandatory with all unexplained deaths) showed nothing physically wrong with the young men. Their hearts were strong; there were no structural abnormalities with their cardiac valves, nor were there problems in their electrical conduction systems. It was a great mystery.

For the Hmong, the deaths were a double tragedy: Not only were they losing their young men to SUDS, the autopsies, which were being performed against their wishes, were condemning the dead men's souls to an eternity of wandering. The Hmong believe that restless souls bring ill health and misfortune to their families for generations to come. Word quickly traveled through the refugee information pipeline, as far away as the Ban Vinai refugee camp in Thailand, where the Hmong cautioned refugees not to go to America because "if you die there, they will take your body and cut it up and your soul will escape."

In 1990, two years after Walker joined the International Clinic, a twenty-one-year-old Hmong man was brought into the hospital's emergency room. He had been asleep at his home when he suddenly sat up, cried out,

and collapsed. His family called 911 and the paramedics were able to get advanced cardiac support to him in time to save his life. Walker, who was supervising the hospital service for that month, saw an opportunity to learn why this otherwise healthy young man had had a sudden cardiac arrest and perhaps understand how to prevent such arrests in the future. She wanted to perform every diagnostic test that she could. "I wanted to do an angiogram of his heart, look for blocked arteries, and then do what's called an EP study, where you insert a catheter into the heart and study the heart electrically to look for abnormal heart rhythms," she recalls. "Our theory about SUDS was that there must be an abnormal heart rhythm that causes this sudden death."

Walker explained to the patient, who was clear-headed and lucid, that he did not have a seizure disorder and was not an epileptic. She told him that the problem was in his heart, and that she wanted to diagnose and treat his condition so he would live a long and healthy life. "I thought if we did this electrophysiologic study and found what we call inducible ventricular fibrillation, we could implant an automatic defibrillator," she says. The young man listened to Walker's explanations of the various tests, but refused to have them done. "The reason I had this attack is because I have been called to be a shaman," he told her. "I have had 'drop attacks' since I was a child. They occur when the ancestor spirits enter me. So I know why these are occurring and I am not worried about them, and I don't want to have the studies."

Seeing the disappointment on her face, he added, "Don't worry about it, Dr. Walker. I will come back to you if it happens again and then I will allow you to do these studies." She knew enough about his culture to know that this was the young man's polite way of saying no to any future tests. Temporizing was the way a Hmong refused a Western physician so that the doctor would not lose face.

One night six months later, Walker received a call at home from the head ER nurse at St. Paul–Ramsey Medical Center, telling her that the young Hmong man who had survived the SUDS attack was dead. He had had another cardiac arrest and this time the paramedics weren't able to resuscitate him. Walker's dilemma now was to decide whether she would sign the death certificate, stating that the man had died of Hmong sudden unexplained death syndrome.

As Walker drove the twenty miles to the hospital, she debated with herself about what to do. If she signed the death certificate, there would be no autopsy. If she didn't sign it, an autopsy would be performed. On the one hand, forcing the issue of an autopsy would cause the family to tell the entire Hmong clan, "Don't go to the hospital because Western doctors will not honor our wishes." On the other hand, an autopsy might reveal the cause for SUDS and thus save lives in the future. Before she had driven halfway to St. Paul, Walker decided to respect the family's wishes and sign the death certificate.

The first thing Walker saw when she entered the ER was the dead man lying on a gurney, surrounded by his entire family— parents, grandparents, aunts, uncles, children—who were keening and rubbing his body. The man's uncle came up to Walker and said, "You must sign the death certificate. Don't even think of not signing it. My nephew must not have an autopsy. We came to America for religious freedom, as Hmong people, and this is our religion. We are animists and these are our beliefs. You must honor our religion." The uncle explained the Hmong concept of soul loss, and that for the next three days the family would be performing funeral rites that would help the young man move on to his next life.

Though she had already decided to sign the certificate, Walker says she appreciated hearing the Hmong beliefs explained so passionately by the uncle. "I signed the certificate and that was the end of it," she says.

Doctors now believe that the deaths of seemingly healthy Hmong immigrants result from a combination of factors, including belief in a nightmare spirit, the stress of facing possible cultural annihilation, and the struggle to maintain one's identity as Hmong. The power of the traditional belief in the nightmare, compounded by such factors as the inability of many refugees to practice traditional healing rituals, brings about cataclysmic psychological stress that can result in the deaths of male Hmong refugees from SUDS.

Pat Walker's learning curve after her return from Thailand's Khao I Dang refugee camp in 1988 was not limited to her new position as medical director at the International Clinic. Shortly before Christmas of that year, she received word that Monorom Sok Hang and his brother, Mony, the two Cambodian men she had agreed to sponsor, were due to arrive at the Minneapolis–St. Paul International Airport. Once again, however, Walker was taken by surprise. Instead of two men walking off the plane to meet her, there were three.

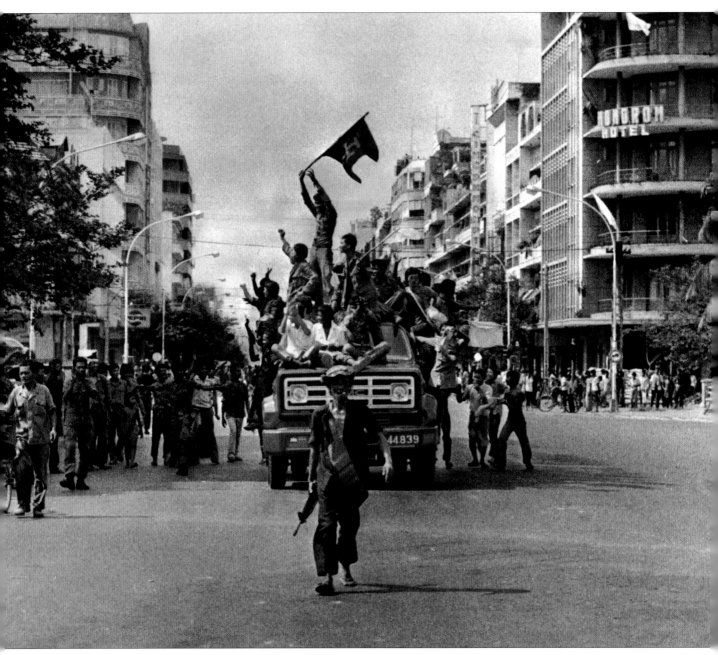

Khmer Rouge troops claim victory in the streets of Phnom Penh on April 17, 1975.

7: Monorom and Mony

THE THIRD CAMBODIAN who accompanied Monorom Sok Hang and his brother, Mony, to the United States was a young medic whom Monica Overkamp, a nurse volunteer with the American Refugee Committee, had agreed to sponsor. The problem was that Overkamp was still in Thailand, and the young man, Soubeth, needed a place to stay until she returned to Minnesota the following year. Pat Walker quickly set up a third bed in her house, bought another parka and set of long underwear, and welcomed all three of the refugees into her home. On the way back from the airport she stopped at an ATM to get each man $20 in cash and to show them how the machines worked. As the dollar bills came streaming out of the ATM, Mony peered around at the back of the machine, certain that there was a man back there feeding in the bills.

Knowing that Asians eat rice at every meal, Walker had purchased a twenty-pound bag, expecting it to last for some time. "It lasted about three days and the boys said, 'Oh no, we are going to starve,'" she remembers. She learned to buy Tabasco sauce in quart bottles. She also heard more of Monorom and Mony's story as, over time, they told her what had happened to them.

On April 17, 1975, seven-year-old Monorom was playing outside his house in Phnom Penh with his six-year-old brother, Mony. Inside were their two older stepsisters and their mother, who was in bed after having given birth to their sister, Rattana, two days before. The quiet of the morning was suddenly shattered when army tanks rumbled onto the family's street. Loudspeakers began broadcasting orders for everyone to vacate the city. The boys' father, the paymaster for the Cambodian army, was in his downtown office. Though his family did not know it, he had probably already been killed.

Soldiers waving rifles burst into their house, warning them that if they did not leave immediately they would be shot. One of Monorom's stepsisters picked up baby Rattana while the other helped their mother out of bed. With the soldiers' bayonets at their backs, they abandoned their home. Monorom clutched Mony's hand and they closely followed their mother and sisters into the confused throng of people on the road. When soldiers fired into the crowd, panicked runners forced themselves between the boys and their mother. The boys tried to keep up but were swept along in the mob that was being forced by the soldiers to the west, out of the city. When the boys were finally able to stop to catch their breath, their mother and sisters were nowhere in sight.

That was at noon. By nightfall the two brothers were standing on the side of the road about ten kilometers outside the city. They were hungry, thirsty, and terrified. All night they stood there, weeping, shouting, and searching the faces in the passing crowd for their mother and sisters. No one stopped to inquire or to care for them as all were running for their lives.

For two days and nights the boys kept their vigil by the side of the road, crying and yelling hour after hour for their mother and sisters. For two days they had nothing to eat or drink. By the end of the second day

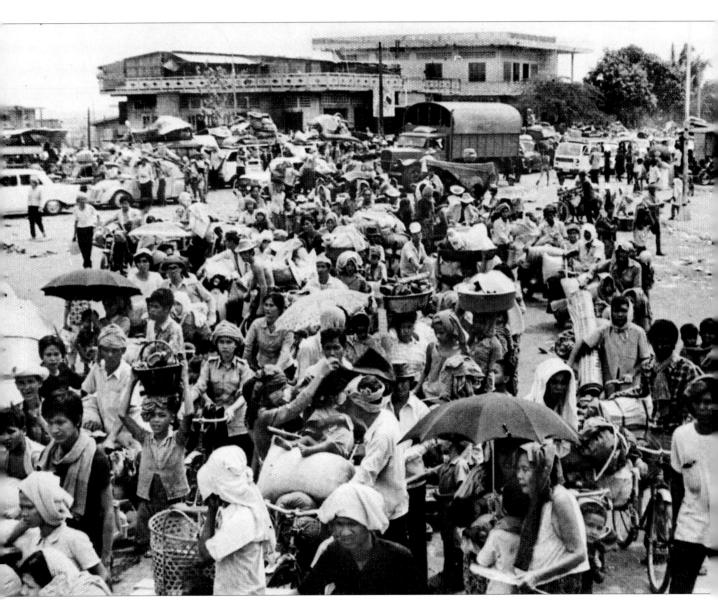

Cambodians flee Phnom Penh after Khmer Rouge troops seized the Cambodian capital.

everyone had fled; no more people came down the road. It was growing dark, and Mony was frantic with thirst and crying. Finding a small plastic cup, Monorom went in search of water for his little brother. He saw, at a distance, a small pond, covered with leaves and grasses and waded in to fill the cup. To his horror, he stepped on a man who was lying face down in the pond. As Monorom cried out in fright, the man, equally startled, rose and clamped his hand over the boy's mouth.

"Shush, shush!" he commanded. As they sat there in the water, the boy in the grasp of the man, the man suddenly relaxed. He recognized Monorom. The man, Veasna, was a colleague of Monorom's father and many times had been a guest in their home. He had been hiding from the soldiers when Monorom discovered him. It was an extraordinary stroke of luck.

"Follow me," Veasna told Monorom, and together with Mony they walked into the jungle.

"We walked day and night," Monorom recalls. "Veasna gave us food because we were starving. He had some cooked and dried rice in his pocket and he gave that to us. He knew survival techniques and I learned a lot from him in the jungle. We ate any kind of living organism we ran into." The three lived on leaves, grasshoppers, crabs, snails, snakes, and lizards. "Veasna delegated the task of finding the food to us," Monorom recalls. "We watched for things to eat at each step. Every animal we could catch we grabbed, killed, and put in our pockets. We collected them along the way until we stopped to rest, when we would make a little fire and cook and eat them."

They climbed trees and slept in the crotches, leaning back against the branches to doze fitfully through the night. Other days Veasna led them across miles of flooded rice fields, where there were no trees in which to hide at night and no dry spots on which to sleep. Veasna showed them how to mound up a pile of mud and muck until it stood a foot above the level of the water. When night fell they rested their heads on the mounds of mud while their bodies floated free in the water. Monorom shudders when he recalls the sleepless nights spent in the chill water. "I was confused from fatigue and from being cold. My hands and feet were numb. We were wet and then dry several times a day."

Veasna was constantly on the alert to avoid being intercepted by the Communist Khmer Rouge. Every time they stopped to rest, he told the boys they had to keep going, that they had to get away, that they were not safe anywhere. "If they catch us, we will die," Veasna warned them. He instructed them to tell anyone who asked that he was their father. He changed his own name to hide his identity and told the boys to change theirs as well. In a Buddhist family a child is given two names: one by the family, which is known as the nickname, and one by the Buddhist monks, which becomes the child's official name, the name used on documents and in school. When Monorom was still a toddler, his father sent him to live for a month with monks and to be given a name that reflected his personality and attitude. The monks named him Monorom, meaning "polite" or "respectful." Monorom used his nickname, La, as his new name.

At one point in their journey the three refugees walked along a road covered with rocks and Mony's feet became bruised and blistered. Monorom tied pieces of cloth torn from his shirt around his brother's feet so he could walk. When that failed, Veasna showed Monorom how to wrap pieces of the fibrous trunk from a banana tree around Mony's feet to form makeshift shoes.

Monorom says that his brother was "crying a lot and I was too." They cried every day, but no longer shed tears; they were too dehydrated. The boys also battled despondency. Monorom was terrified about where they were going, about getting food, about being alone, and about losing his family.

They walked for weeks. To Monorom it seemed that they had walked around the Earth. He now knows that they walked about 150 miles, to a town Veasna knew. They arrived just as the Khmer Rouge were evacuating the town, so they trudged another six miles to an abandoned rice field, where they built a small hut. Monorom and Mony lived in the hut with Veasna for four or five months before they were discovered by Khmer Rouge soldiers, who took the boys away from Veasna to live in a children's mobile team work camp.

The Khmer Rouge put boys into their various camps according to age. To determine younger from older children, "they had us put our arm around our head, and if our hand could reach to the other side of our head to our ear, we were old enough to be in the children's team," explains Monorom. "You were supposed to be seven years old and older. I was about eight by now and my brother was close to seven." The soldiers sent the brothers to separate work camps.

For Monorom, life in the camp was the worst of his experiences, like being in a jail with no walls. "We could see open space, but could not go there," he remembers. About two hundred boys lived in a shelter that was more an open sewer than a dwelling, and slept head to toe on the ground. There were no sanitary facilities or latrines. "The children lived in unspeakable filth," Monorom says. "We were kept worse than animals."

The boys worked from four or five in the morning until six or seven at night. They were ordered to flatten a two-hundred-foot-high hill with their bare hands to make it suitable for planting rice. They used sticks to pry rocks from the ground. They became living scarecrows, running round and round rice paddies, hour after hour, to scare away foraging birds. Weeding the rice paddies enabled them to survive. "That is how we got things to eat," Monorom says. "We ate the snails and crabs in the water."

When crops were ready for harvest, the boys were told they each had to kill one hundred rats a day and bring the heads into the camp or they would be punished. They dug holes in the ground to catch the rats. When Monorom's best friend put his hand into a hole, he was bitten by a cobra. Two or three minutes later the boy was short of breath and turned blue. Monorom picked up his friend and began to carry him toward the village for help, but the boy died before he could get there. Monorom witnessed many other deaths, he says, "but that was the one that got to me the most."

Every night the boys were forced to listen to disciplinary lectures as soldiers beat and tormented those who hadn't followed orders. "If you don't obey us, this is what will happen to you," the guards warned them. "The boys would have trouble keeping awake during the lectures," Monorom remembers. "Children tried to escape, and when they were caught they were terribly punished." They were beaten, flayed with horse whips, starved, or tied to stakes, defenseless against the stinging ants that were placed on their bodies. "Children died every day from illness and starvation," Monorom says. "I can still close my eyes and see it all."

Monorom and Mony survived four torturous years in separate camps until the Vietnamese invasion drove out the Khmer Rouge. In the resulting chaos, the brothers escaped and made their way to the town where they found Veasna, whom they thought of as their adopted father.

For the next few years the adolescent Mono survived by smuggling. Because there was no currency in Cambodia, rice and gold had become the medium of exchange. A Cambodian would give Mono some grams of gold for him to carry into Thailand, where he would buy and bring back sugar and cigarettes. It was a hazardous trip as he evaded land mines, Vietnamese patrols, and border guards. He knew it was only a matter of time before he would be caught and killed. Besides, a successful smuggler had to be a big man, strong enough to carry large quantities of goods—forty pounds of sugar and twenty pairs of shoes—and to fend off robbers. Mono stood only five feet, three inches tall and weighed less than one hundred

pounds. After surviving two smuggling trips from Cambodia into Thailand and back, Monorom and his brother decided to find another way to stay alive. They hid in Thailand and began to smuggle goods and people from the Thai border into the Khao I Dang refugee camp.

"Khao I Dang was a camp guarded by Thai soldiers," Monorom explains. "Those people who lived inside the camp could not get out to get things they needed and wanted. So we bribed the Thai guards. We would say, 'Meet us at 2:00 a.m. I will be here. I will bring you this amount of gold and you let us through.' Ten grams of gold would get one person in."

Going in and out of Khao I Dang on his smuggling expeditions, Mono began to learn about the camp: that the United Nations ran the camp to help refugees, to provide food and perhaps a chance for some education, even the possibility of settling in another country. Though the camp consisted of one square mile that was surrounded by fences patrolled by armed soldiers, it looked to Monorom like a safe place to stay. He decided to bribe his way in again and this time he would stay. He was seventeen years old.

Like Veera and Channy Som, the two sisters Pat Walker had met during her year in Thailand, Monorom was an "illegal" refugee. The only way he could get something to eat was to beg for leftover food that had been given to patients in the hospital who were too sick to eat it all. After a few months Monorom managed to change his status to "legal" and decided that he should repay the hospital for its food by working there. He took the ARC course in basic health and became a camp health educator. Because he had no money for the English classes offered in the camp, he stood outside the classroom shelter, listening and trying to learn. "They kept chasing me away," he remembers, but he persevered. "I would peek through the blinds at the words written on a chalkboard."

When Monorom qualified to become a medic, he began working one day a week with Khao I Dang's medical director, Pat Walker. "I did translating, got the history from the patient, wrote simple prescriptions for pain killers," he says. "Pat began to ask me questions, and when we got to know each other, I shared some of my personal life with her."

Monorom remembers the moment when Walker told him that she would try to help him. Almost two decades later, Monorom still cannot tell the story without weeping: "Just hearing that one word 'help'—I will try not to cry—I did not know what she meant. . . . I longed to hear the word 'help' from my boss, from a foreigner, from an American. That word made me change my way of

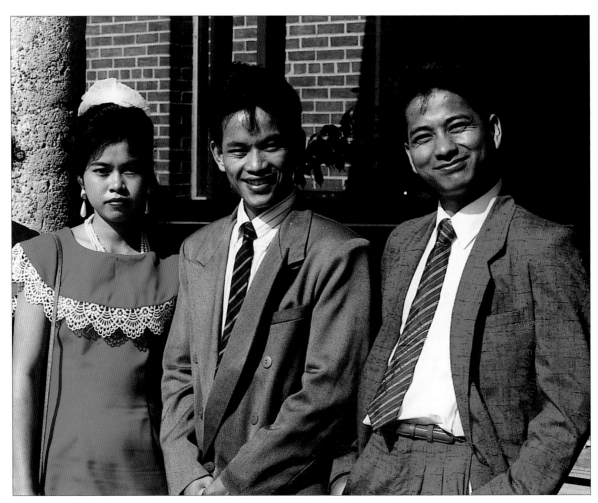

Rattana, Monorom, and Mony Hang at a Cambodian wedding, soon after Rattana was reunited with her brothers in Minneapolis.

thinking, change my life. I was never afraid of death. I could run across the mined border with the patrol shooting at me without fear. But when she said she would help me, it changed my feeling, my plan, my everything. I started to dream. My dream was to get away and find a place for myself."

After Monorom and Mony arrived in the United States in 1988, Monorom contacted the Red Cross for help in locating his mother and sister Rattana, whom he had not seen since the day they were separated while fleeing Phnom Penh in 1975. The Red Cross was unsuccessful, but his "foster father" Veasna, who knew all about Monorom's family, eventually found both his mother and young sister. Monorom tried to arrange to speak with his mother, and rushed money to her, but she died soon after receiving it. They never spoke, but "before she died, my mother learned that her two boys had survived," Monorom says.

In 1991, with help from Walker and immigration attorney Glenda Potter, Monorom sponsored his sixteen-year-old sister Rattana, whom he had last seen when she was two days old, to come to the United States. She too moved in with Pat Walker and her partner. "I cannot find a word to describe how thankful I am to Pat," Monorom says. "I was raised without anybody to give me advice; I learned by observing people. No one, before Pat, gave me support."

Within weeks of his arrival in the United States, Monorom found a job in the International Clinic at St. Paul–Ramsey Medical Center as a Cambodian interpreter. He worked there for two years before he realized that his job provided benefits and days off.

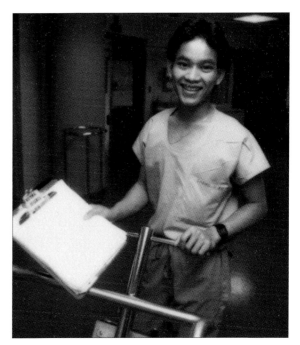

In 1996 Monorom Hang graduated as a registered nurse from Century College in White Bear Lake, Minnesota, and landed a job at Regions Hospital in St. Paul.

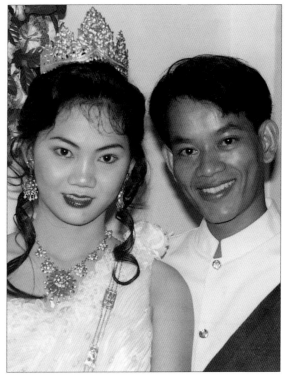

Monorom and his wife, Naroeun, on their wedding day.

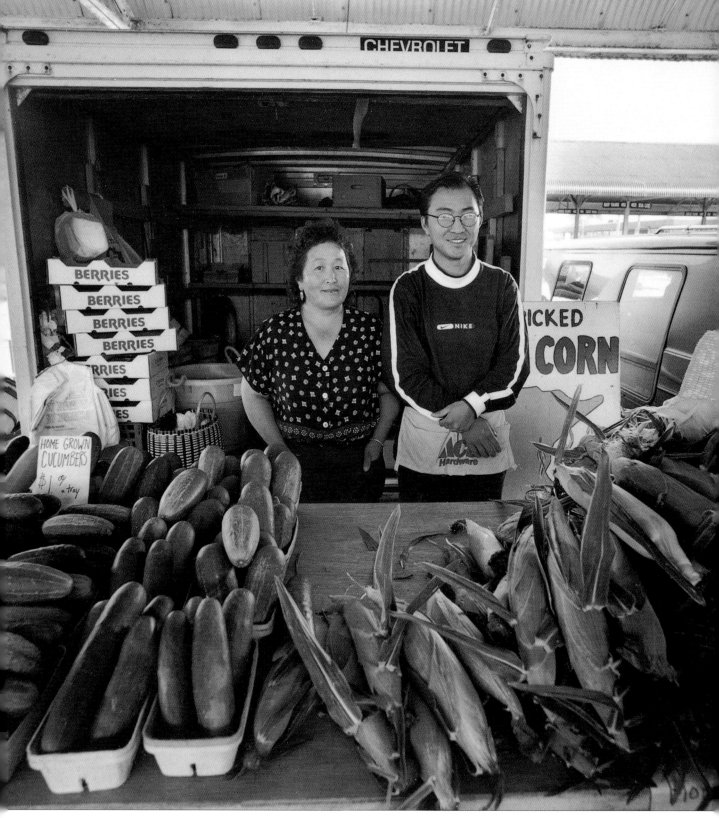

Mother and son Keu and Sao Vang from Hugo, Minnesota, at the Minneapolis Farmers' Market in 1998. Many Hmong in Minnesota farm small rented plots where they grow corn as well as traditional vegetables such as cucumbers and peppers in their time-honored ways, planting and hoeing and reaping by hand. Farmers' markets provide an outlet for their produce.

8: interpreters wanted

BY 1991, MINNESOTA had become a magnet for refugees, in large part because local churches and four Twin Cities–based social service agencies had extended helping hands. The people working at Lutheran Social Services, Catholic Charities, Jewish Family Services, and the International Institute of Minnesota were committed to making a difference in human lives, with the result that the number of refugees coming to Minnesota was higher than in most other states.

More than three thousand patients a year were finding their way into the waiting room of the International Clinic at St. Paul–Ramsey Medical Center. With the growing demand for the more specialized health services the clinic offered, medical director Pat Walker was anxious to find more interpreters. With a grant from the State of Minnesota Refugee and Immigrant Assistance Division of the Department of Human Services, she hired four new interpreters, doubling the translator staff. When the one-year grant ran out, hospital administrator and CEO Jim Dixon put the interpreters on the St. Paul–Ramsey payroll. Though they spent most of their time in the International Clinic, they also worked in other departments throughout the hospital. "That is the

wonderful glue of the interpreters," Walker explains. "They are in the emergency room, in surgery, everywhere. If I send a patient to a cardiologist, the same interpreter goes with him."

Dixon strongly supported the International Clinic, informed, in part, by his experience of attending a Hmong funeral at the invitation of family practitioner Kathleen Culhane-Pera. He, a tall white man, found himself in a room filled with short Asian men. He felt acutely uncomfortable in the minority and realized for the first time how immigrant patients must feel when they come into the hospital. That singular experience shifted Dixon's thinking about how St. Paul–Ramsey and the International Clinic should care for people from different cultures.

Many of the hospital's physicians also now embraced, or at least recognized the need for, the work of the clinic. A colleague who ran the geriatric clinic across the hallway from the International Clinic said to Walker, "I saw one of your people who was sent to me because of his age. I don't want to see him. I don't know what I am doing with him. You guys do a much better job, so I'm going to send him back to you."

For other physicians, immigrant patients remained a bother: "Why don't they learn to speak English? Why can't they understand the Western medical system?" When twenty relatives would crowd around a Hmong patient in an intensive care unit, a doctor's response, not always spoken, was, "Get out. We can't do our work with so many people here." Some staff applied different standards to different patients. When a Christian Science follower refused to have a blood transfusion, his physician might say, "All right. It's the patient's religion." But when a Hmong animist would say, "Don't cut into me because of soul loss," the same doctor might think the patient was crazy.

Some of these attitudes at the hospital changed after Walker received a call from the International Organization for Migration, based in Geneva, Switzerland. She was known to the organization because of her work at the Khao I Dang refugee camp, where she was responsible for selecting medically at-risk cases to send abroad for specialized treatment. The caller from Geneva asked Walker if her hospital would be willing to take in and treat, at no charge, Nikola Brkic, a young man from Bosnia-Herzegovina who had badly injured his leg stepping on a land mine.

St. Paul–Ramsey administrator Jim Dixon agreed to the surgery, which was performed by orthopedic surgeon Dan Gaither. The hospital donated nursing and physical therapy services as well as medications. Local newspapers covered the story and everyone involved with Brkic's care felt wonderful about what they had done. "This is the reason we are here at this hospital," they told themselves. But as feelings of self-satisfaction and congratulation washed over the hospital, many staff still felt vaguely guilty about the negative attitudes toward immigrants that surfaced from time to time in their institution. Despite their frustrations with the immigrant patients, the staff had good hearts. They knew that their impatience came from not understanding the new cultures that were moving into Minnesota and causing profound changes in their workplace.

A Cross-Cultural Supervisor

Aware that the International Clinic was stretched thin and close to being overwhelmed by issues related to the immigrant community, Dixon organized a Southeast Asian Task Force to find ways for St. Paul–Ramsey to provide better health care to its immigrant patients. After a year's study, the task force recommended that the hospital hire more interpreters, as well as a cross-cultural supervisor who would manage the interpreters and any immigrant concerns as they arose.

By coincidence, Pat Walker's sister, Elizabeth Anderson, and her husband, Jim, had returned from Bangkok and were working for the Joint Volunteer Agency in Chicago, adjudicating political asylum cases. Both wanted to return to Minnesota, so Pat called Elizabeth about the new supervisory position. Rebecca Enos, chief nursing officer for St. Paul–Ramsey, had no idea that Elizabeth was Pat's sister until she put two and two together while reading her application resume. Enos hired Elizabeth in January 1992 to oversee the staff of twelve full-time interpreters (and as many as thirty-five temporary translators) and to encourage

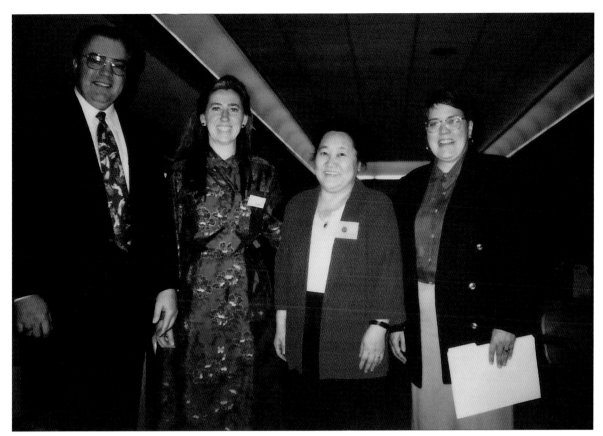

Jim Dixon, president and CEO of St. Paul–Ramsey Medical Center; Elizabeth Walker Anderson, director of interpreter services; Xiong My Ly, who received the "Pro of the Month" award; and Becky Enos, senior vice president for patient care services.

physicians to use interpreters when communicating with their non–English-speaking patients. Demand for in-house lectures on cross-cultural issues with Southeast Asians began to come in faster than Anderson could deal with them.

Anderson's task was not always easy. She remembers going into the room of a Hmong patient and learning that the staff had not called for an interpreter. "I asked the doctor how he could understand what the patient's symptoms were so he could properly diagnose and treat him. 'Well,' the doctor replied, 'he understands if I gesture. He is hot, has a fever, and points to where he hurts.'"

Anderson was stunned that intelligent medical professionals could not see the value of having linguistic and cultural connections to their patients. How would they otherwise understand that such customs as "coining"—the Cambodian practice of vigorously rubbing a coin on the skin—was not abuse, but a parent's effort to bring out the fever in a child? Anderson's challenge was to find ways to educate physicians without impugning their medical knowledge.

"Doctors do not like the idea of having to go through an interpreter or having their prescriptions translated into another language," she explains. "It is just more work to take care of people who are different

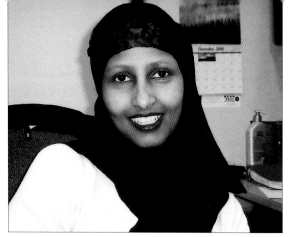

Somali interpreter Fartun Wardere fled Mogadishu with her family to a refugee camp in Kenya when civil war erupted in Somalia.

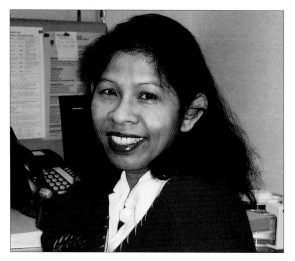

Cambodian interpreter Channy Som and her sister Veera survived two refugee camps in Thailand before coming here in 1990.

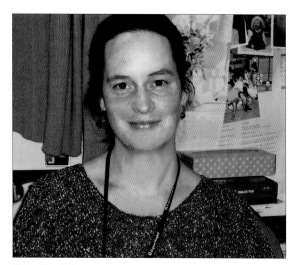

Sidney Van Dyke speaks Indonesian and French, and now oversees interpreters for five Health Partners sites in addition to CIH.

from you. There was definitely always a barrier. Medicine has its own culture. I understood the problems refugees faced dealing with the American medical culture, along with their own issues about how they wanted to have health care delivered. It helped a lot that my supervisor, Rebecca Enos, had been reared in Africa and was a missionary kid."

With the clinic's non–English-speaking patient population growing, Anderson advertised for more interpreters through the hospital's human resources department, stating as a minimum qualification fluency in Vietnamese and English and six months' experience in a medical setting. She got applicants, but none were suitable. "Their language abilities were not good and they had no clue what the medical world was like," she says. Running out of options, she called her friends at Lutheran Social Services and explained her problem, saying, "Our patients deserve a better interpreter than the candidates I have been seeing."

The agency promised to help and sent over multiple candidates for the position. But they were not passed on to Anderson for interviews because they had not made it past human resources' screening. In frustration, she asked the HR department to send her every person who applied.

"But that is not our system," the staff replied.

"I don't care what our system is," Anderson said. "We are not getting the right caliber of individuals in here. Send me everyone."

That is how she got Diem Ngoc Nguyen. A slim, dignified, exceptionally well-spoken man who had been rejected by HR for an interpreter position, Diem Nguyen walked into Anderson's office one day in 1994. When she asked him why he was interested in being an interpreter, he replied, "I was in prison for many years and I know the heartache of many of my fellow countrymen. I think I can make a contribution here." The former diplomat and teacher had been abroad when South Vietnam fell. "I came back because I felt I owed it to my country," he said. "That is when I was thrown into the prison camp."

Diem spoke French and English as well as Vietnamese. He had learned a great deal about medicine from his fellow prisoners, physicians who had conducted lessons on diseases of the body and mind to pass the time. "I am writing a medical dictionary in French, Vietnamese, and English," Diem added. "My daughter is doing the illustrations." When he mentioned that in Vietnamese the word "hospital" means "house of love," Anderson hired him.

People soon began raving to her about Diem. "It wasn't just his intellectual capacity and his kind nature," she says. "He would work all through his lunch hour, stay as late as we needed him, quietly help patients behind the scenes." One of the physicians reported to her that a Vietnamese patient was brought into the emergency room with heart failure and the staff could not find the man's chart. Diem, who was on duty to interpret, recited the patient's entire medical history from memory for the doctor.

"How do you know this?" the doctor asked.

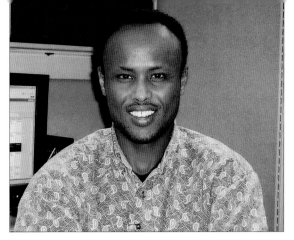

Somali interpreter Mohamud Aden came to the U.S. in 1991. His coworkers enjoy his sense of humor.

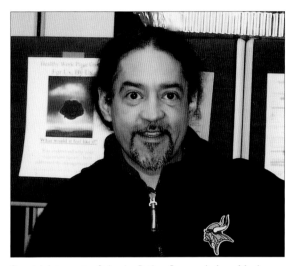

Spanish interpreter Salvador Patino-Guzman is from Mexico. He is both a father and a grandfather.

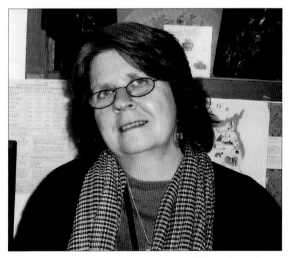

Spanish interpreter Kathy Jenkins worked with Cesar Chavez in California and migrant farm workers in the Midwest.

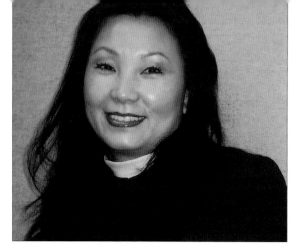

Head interpreter Shelly Daohevang (who speaks Hmong and Lao) came to the U.S. in 1980 when she was eight years old.

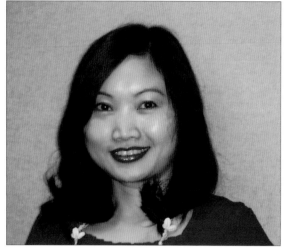

Vietnamese interpreter Danglan Nguyen is married and has a two-year-old son. She came to the U.S. in 2001.

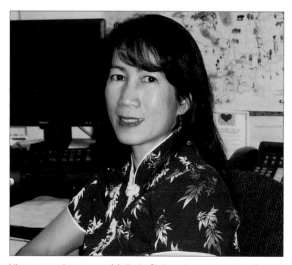

Vietnamese interpreter Malinda Christopher also speaks Cambodian. She is married and has two children.

"I remember him from the clinic," Diem replied.

Diem was always careful to respect the boundary between physician and interpreter, but he also knew when to cross that line when it benefited both the physician and patient. Although he was careful not to disclose information that a patient had not freely offered, Diem made sure that the doctors for whom he interpreted understood a little of what their patients had experienced in their lives. "After the doctors finished examining their patients, I always added something so that they will know more about their patients. Once you know what has happened to them, you can never forget. Then the patients cease to be medical cases and become people—human beings."

"The thing about Diem and the other interpreters at the hospital is that they are the true primary-care providers," Anderson says. "They are the ones who follow the patient from billing to parking-lot issues, to meetings with the doctors, to the emergency department, to inpatient and outpatient work. It is part of their duties. Every place the patient touches the health-care system, the interpreter is there. As a result, strong relationships build up that are often far more intense than those between the physician and the patient because the interpreter is a person of his own culture."

One day in 1995, Dr. Eric Egli, a psychologist who was working at the International Clinic, asked Anderson to assign Diem as a permanent interpreter for a weekly therapy group of Vietnamese men that Egli had organized. All of them had been held in prison camps in Vietnam. Though he was on duty as the group's interpreter, Diem was also a participant. It was a great success, even after Egli moved on and a Russian immigrant psychologist, Georgi Kroupin, took over. Anderson credits Diem with much of that success. "They had great rapport with each other," she says. "Diem did simultaneous interpreting, and they felt comfortable talking with him. They trusted him."

Diem can never forget the stories of his fellow interpreters or the patients they served. "When you know them longer, you learn that each has a long story to tell." As he ticks off their names, it's evident that he became their confidante. "There is Malinda. She is one of the Vietnamese-Cambodian interpreters. Her father was Chinese, her mother from Vietnam, but they lived in Cambodia. One day the Khmer Rouge came and horrible things happened to them. She crossed the sea and came here. Other Cambodian interpreters lost their siblings or their children were killed. The father of another interpreter, a colonel of paratroopers, spent ten years in jail."

Diem recalls the story of a patient who was the daughter of a former district chief in Vietnam, a position that is similar to that of a state's governor. The family was sitting down to dinner one evening when the patient, at the time a girl of ten, excused herself to use the outdoor bathroom. During her absence the Communists broke into her home and killed everyone. The girl was reared by an aunt, and when she was grown the girl married a young man who had been a student of Diem's. That young man later spent ten years in prison.

Diem's own story of imprisonment covered twelve horrific years.

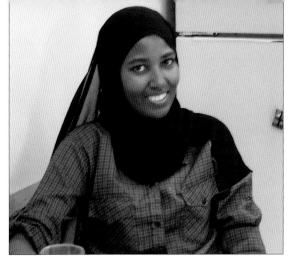

Oromo interpreter Mardiya Jaffer emigrated with her family from Addis Ababa, Ethiopia, in 1995.

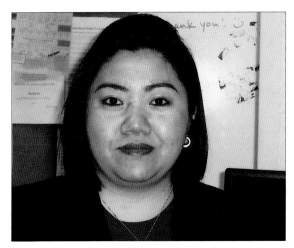

Hmong and Lao interpreter Soua Her came to the U.S. in 1979. She is married and has four children.

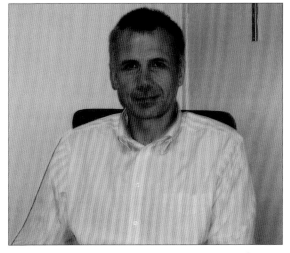

Russian Georgi Kroupin is the lead psychologist for the Center for International Health.

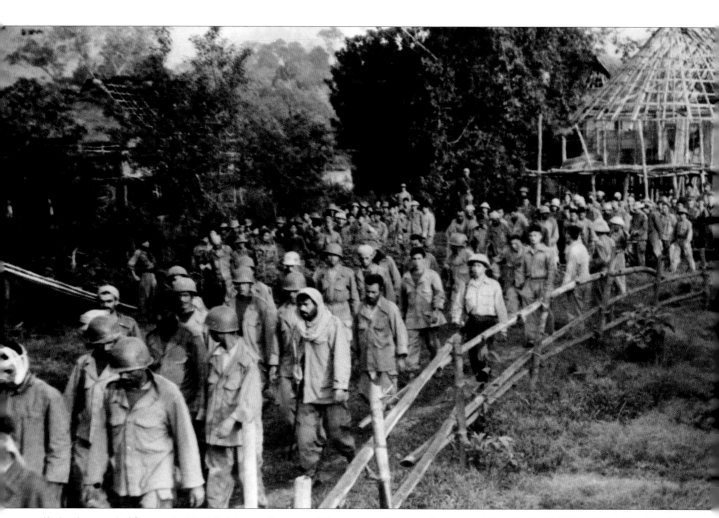

Under the guard of Communist Viet Minh troops, French and Vietnamese prisoners of war march from the battlefields of Dien Bien Phu. The 1954 battle of Dien Bien Phu marked the fall of French Indochina.

9: Diem Ngoc Nguyen

IN ALL OF HIS IMAGININGS, it never crossed Diem Nguyen's mind that he would some-day become an interpreter in an American hospital. When he lived in Vietnam, his goal in life had been to earn his doctorate in French literature and to teach.

Born in 1936 in North Vietnam to Buddhist parents, young Diem attended Tpuginier, a Catholic school run by the French Brothers of Saint Jean de Baptiste de la Salle. The order taught the sons of the poor, who received an excellent education for very little tuition. "My father did not have any objection for me attending a Catholic school," Nguyen remembers. "He did not mind about religion. 'Buddhists and Catholics are all good,' he said. What he could not tolerate was Communism. He said that Communism is atheistic and does not allow one to think individually. My teachers were humble men and good teachers. We had Catechism for fifteen minutes every morning, but they never tried to force religion on us.

"We had to take two foreign languages. Since French was considered the native language, I took Vietnamese as my first foreign language and English for my second. I was a top student. During my exams I slept only five hours a night and studied the rest of

the time. I got my French baccalaureate in 1954."

For a century Vietnam had been occupied by the French, who had established the first university in Indochina at Hanoi. "No true Vietnamese liked the French occupation," Nguyen recalls. "While they understood the

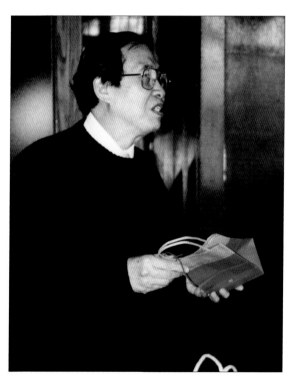

Diem Ngoc Nguyen, former director of European and Middle East affairs for South Vietnam and later interpreter for the Center for International Health.

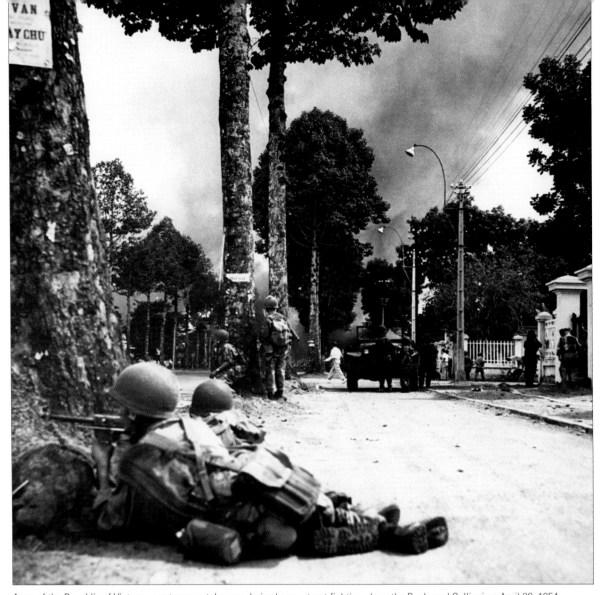

Army of the Republic of Vietnam paratroopers take over during heavy street fighting along the Boulevard Gallieni on April 28, 1954.

benefits the French brought to Vietnam, and through the French the exposure to Western civilization, they did not like the French presence."

Colonial rule ended following France's defeat at the battle of Dien Bien Phu in May 1954. The Geneva Accords divided Vietnam at the 17th Parallel, placing North Vietnam under Communist rule and South Vietnam under the anti-Communist leadership of Prime Minister Ngo Dinh Diem. The division represented the worst of all possible futures for Vietnam. When the country was

divided, Diem Nguyen's widowed mother decided to leave everything in the North—her home, possessions, and business—and move her family of seven children to the South. About a million other North Vietnamese did the same.

Fearing persecution, the Catholic brothers closed their school and also prepared to move to the South. "Our teachers talked to us and said, 'If you want to go, we will take you.' My mother said, 'You go first and we will come later.' So I followed my teachers." Almost the entire population of

Nguyen's school sailed on a large Swedish ship to the South. The voyage took four days. "When my teachers brought me to Saigon, my uncle, who was a captain in the ministry of defense, met me. My teachers turned me over to him and said that they had now discharged their responsibility. I had never been away from home before. I was eighteen years old."

Nguyen moved in with his uncle and family and enrolled in the University of Saigon. At the end of two years he had earned certificates in French civilization and French literature and was teaching at Chu Van An, the most prestigious high school in Saigon. The following year he earned two more certificates, for which he had to learn Chinese characters. In his last year at the university he took certificates in Vietnamese history and the history of Southeast Asia, impressive and advanced academic credentials.

By the early 1960s Nguyen was teaching full-time, had bought a house for his mother and siblings, was courting his future wife, and had become a judge and an examiner of the South Vietnamese schools. As his reputation in the scholarly community spread, he continued to dream of the day when he would study French literature at a university in Paris and earn his doctorate. "My wish was to go abroad and become a teacher at the highest level," he recalls.

While Nguyen's life and career as a teacher was making rapid progress, the political situation in South Vietnam was not. Prime Minister Diem, whose brother was the country's Roman Catholic archbishop, had begun persecuting the Buddhists, who represented 95 percent of the population, claiming they had been infiltrated by Communists.

It was not long before Nguyen felt this prejudice personally. A French university offered him a full scholarship to go to France for two years to study for his doctorate, but the South Vietnamese government refused to let him go, saying he had enough degrees. Then a friend of his, a man who was less qualified but who happened to be a member of the Catholic faith, was offered the same scholarship and allowed to go. "I felt it was not fair," Nguyen says. A few months later he was again offered the French scholarship, the only one given in all of South Vietnam, but again the government refused Nguyen permission to leave.

Becoming a Diplomat

Shortly after Nguyen's wedding in 1963, the prime minister of South Vietnam and his brother were overthrown in a coup and assassinated. Two years later, Nguyen spotted a notice in the newspaper that the government was giving its first competitive examinations to recruit individuals for the foreign ministry. "Before, it was a closed system, and relatives of officials were the only ones named," he says. "I did not have any clue as to what the job would be like, [but] I wanted to join the ministry just for the opportunity to go abroad and complete my studies."

The examination was in two parts, written and oral. "We did not know the topic in advance," Nguyen says of the written exam. His subject was "Diplomatic Relationships between Vietnam, Cambodia, and Laos in the Past and Present." One week later he took the oral exam. Nineteen of the forty exam candidates were chosen, including Nguyen, who was sent to the most difficult diplomatic post in Indochina: Vientiane, the capital of Laos. He moved there with his wife, Thu, and their one-year-old son and two-year-old daughter. Nguyen was also drafted into the military. "Teachers in Vietnam were the only civil servants who were exempt from the draft," he explains. "You got a deferment if you were a teacher because education is number one in Vietnam. For Vietnamese, knowledge always trumps everything and academic degrees imply some kind of morality. I got drafted only when I became a diplomat."

A hotbed of spies and intrigue, Vientiane was home to the embassies of South and North Vietnam, the Soviet Union, China, and the United States. Nguyen became acquainted with Joseph G. Sullivan, the U.S. ambassador who was running America's secret war in Laos, and learned that the North Vietnamese were violating the sovereignty of Laos by infiltrating through the mountains on the Ho Chi Min Trail to get into South Vietnam. And Nguyen also got to know Vang Pao, the Hmong general of the Lao army who was governor of the Second Military Zone. "He spoke three languages and was a sophisticated man," Nguyen remembers. "He was a very good general, part of the loyal Lao army."

Nguyen says he lived by the code of the diplomat: "People at the time did not talk about the violation of the borders. . . . Sometimes they asked you for things that you could not talk about. But a diplomat never lies. Never! If you lie, it is finished. If they ask you something and you do not want to talk about it, you just do not say anything. . . .

But if you do say something, it must be the truth. If you ask someone something and he smiles but does not say anything, you respect that and never push. This was the code of the diplomatic powers in the free world. In other countries, if you were a diplomat, you could be (and probably were) a spy. Ninety percent of the North Vietnam diplomats were spies. They were trained to be spies, but I was not."

In 1967, while Nguyen was in Laos, two men from the Rand Corporation, a California thinktank, visited the American embassy and Nguyen was among a small group invited to talk with them. At that time, the U.S. government was bombing North Vietnam, as well as the infiltration route through Laos. At the meeting someone asked the Rand visitors if they thought the bombing would be effective.

"Very carefully they said, 'We do not believe the bombing will be successful.' I was young and asked why. They explained that if North Vietnam were an industrial country, the bombing would be useful because it would destroy electrical grids and power plants. But North Vietnam was rural. 'How can we win bombing water buffalo?' they asked. I sent this report back to South Vietnam, but I do not know what they did with it.

"When you know all about these things and when things are not encouraging, you feel disappointed. I always believed in our final success. I did not believe South Vietnam would be conquered. . . . It is why I was later so disappointed. If you did not have much faith, you were not disappointed. But I was a believer."

In February 1968, the North Vietnamese launched the Tet Offensive and Nguyen was recalled to Saigon. When the Paris peace talks began, he was part of a small group in the foreign ministry that provided support and information to the South Vietnamese delegation in Paris. He was then posted to Manila, where he was first secretary of the embassy in charge of consular affairs. At the end of four years, he was called back to Saigon and named director of European and Middle East affairs, directly under the foreign minister. The situation in South Vietnam had worsened and government officials could see that the country was collapsing. When the U.S. Congress re-fused to supply further aid, Saudi Arabia expressed interest in providing funds, so Nguyen, the foreign minister, and the minister of economic affairs flew to Saudi Arabia in a last-ditch effort to seek help. For three days they presented their case to King Khalid and Prince Fahd. Their mission was unsuccessful.

As the three men prepared to depart the Riyadh airport, the South Vietnamese foreign minister was suddenly called to Washington, D.C. Only the minister of economic affairs and Nguyen flew on to Saigon. The foreign minister's abrupt departure troubled Nguyen because he did not believe it was in the man's nature to abandon his country.

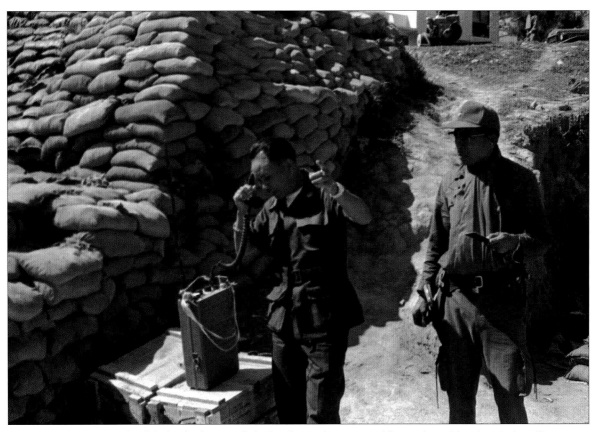

General Vang Pao, commander of the Laotian forces, calls in air strikes against suspected Communist positions from the Long Chen command post in January 1972. CIA agents had become accustomed to operating unfettered by the scrutiny of the American public, but now for the first time in its ten-year history journalists were admitted and given free access to the base.

For years Nguyen was to wonder if he had misjudged the foreign minister's character.

On April 14, 1975, Nguyen's plane touched down for a stopover at Bangkok and he telephoned his office. When his colleague said, "Enjoy your last trip out of the country," he knew that it was the end. In full knowledge that their government was collapsing and that they faced certain imprisonment, Nguyen and the minister of economic affairs flew home to South Vietnam. Nguyen returned to his office in the foreign ministry on April 15 to receive courtesy calls of diplomats who were leaving the country. The chargé d'affaires of Canada and the ambassadors of Germany and the Netherlands all came to say farewell and good luck to Nguyen. "It was like people leaving a sinking ship. They knew everything and I knew everything, but we did not discuss it." The personnel of only two embassies, the French and the American, stayed on until the end.

The staff at the foreign ministry continued to hold its scheduled morning meetings, though attendance kept dropping. Everyone knew that some senior government officials had fled the country while others stayed. South Vietnam fell on April 30 and the next day Nguyen went to his office as usual. One of the secretaries saw him and exclaimed, "We thought you had abandoned us!" "Never!" he said. "That is why I came back." The Viet Cong quickly occupied the building and told Nguyen to go home and listen to his radio for orders.

Imprisonment

Within a few days Nguyen was told to report to an orphanage outside Saigon where, with one thousand others, he was confined for a year. The prisoners were then loaded into the hold of a ship bound for Haiphong in North Vietnam. "We were like animals, packed in," he recalls. "They put food in a huge bucket and lowered it down to us. And we had to defecate in the same bucket." The voyage lasted four days and three nights. When they disembarked, Nguyen and the others were taken to a prison camp very close to the Chinese border in the north. The men were put to work growing potatoes, rice, and tapioca. Their only food was thirty pounds of rice each for a month. The prisoners were cold and hungry all of the time. "You lose weight, a little bit, every day. And then your immune system becomes so weak that you die from simple diseases like dysentery. People died, died, died. I had a friend who spent his free time writing recipes on tiny pieces of paper to keep his hunger at bay." Despite their misery, the prisoners would not let on to their guards that they were distressed.

"The men in the camp were the intellectuals of South Vietnam," Nguyen says. "We had doctors, lawyers, priests, generals, writers, pharmacists, diplomats. They were all educated people. My education helped me a lot. I thought of Pascal, Descartes—'I think, therefore I am.' The more I think, the more I exist. I liked Pascal very much. He said that we are like a reed, but because of our mind, we can visualize the world. . . .

"When people learned I was a teacher, they came to me and asked me many questions. In the winter, when we could not sleep for the cold, we sat up and I told stories. I talked about the books *Crime and Punishment* and *Brothers Karamazov*. I like

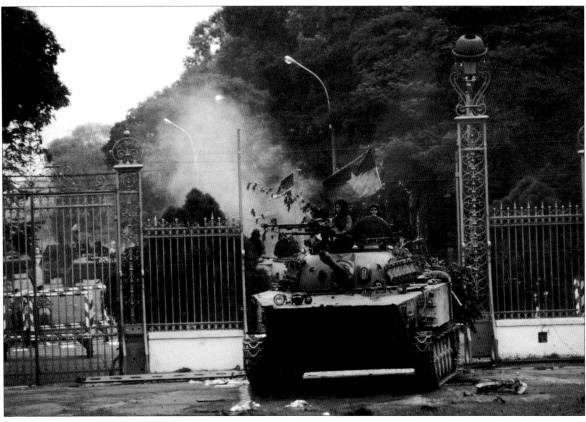

A North Vietnamese tank breaks through the gates to the presidential palace in Saigon on April 30, 1975. Saigon surrendered the next day, ending the United States' fifteen-year involvement in Vietnam.

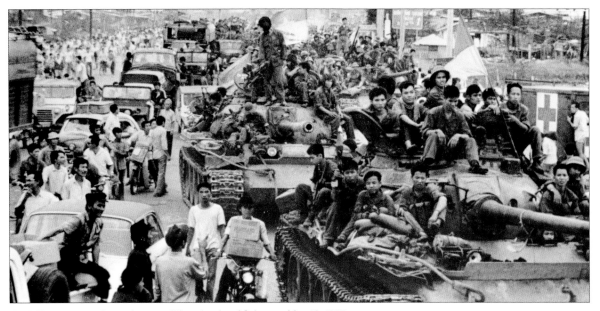

North Vietnamese tanks continue to roll into the city of Saigon on May 12, 1975.

Dostoyevsky very much. I told them that suffering must have a meaning, that we have to find out the meaning of our suffering here. I tried to tell them stories and stimulate their minds to help them forget their misery, their cold, and their stomachs." Nguyen, who had never written poetry before his time in jail, began to compose verses. "Since I had no paper at that time, I memorized the ones I composed and tried to force my mind on something other than my stomach."

Two years into Nguyen's imprisonment, events on the international scene again affected his life. China attacked North Vietnam, its former ally. The initial attack took place very near the prison camp, so the inmates were taken to another camp, this one deep in the jungle. As the trucks neared the new camp, they stopped at a poor hut at the edge of the forest where two sisters sold bananas, sugar cane, and tea to passers-by. After the guards ate and drank, the sisters brought stalks of sugar cane to the prisoners.

"Because I was born in North Vietnam, I knew how poor the people were and I refused the gift of cane," Nguyen recalls. "One of my Buddhist friends told me (and this is one of the great lessons I received when I was in jail) that to complete an act of charity you must have a donor and a receiver. 'If you refuse to accept the gift, you do not help these women achieve an act of charity.' In a moment I saw the problem. Very humbly I turned to the woman and accepted."

If the old camp was bad, the next one was worse. Prisoners slept on the ground, with only a thatched roof over them. There was no electricity. Their diet consisted of rice, potatoes, and tapioca. The prisoners were allowed one fifteen-minute visit a year from family members. When Nguyen's wife and children came to see him in 1979, the couple was directed to sit on opposite sides of a table with a guard between them. The children stood behind their mother. They were not allowed to touch, but as her visit was ending, Nguyen's wife suddenly leaned forward and quickly passed him two bits of information. One was that she had visited a noted Buddhist priest, who agreed to her request to accept Nguyen as an acolyte and gave him his Buddhist name. The other was that the U.S. government was working to negotiate the release of political prisoners.

The news of his wife's visit to the Buddhist priest cheered Nguyen. "I was born into a Buddhist family, but I rarely went to the temple," he says. "But when we were in jail, I had time to think about many things. When I received the formal Buddhist name, I felt that I belonged to my religion and started to talk about it with my friends who knew more than I. Many Buddhist priests, Catholic priests, and Protestant ministers were in the jail. One was a Buddhist who had been a professor at the university in South Vietnam. He spoke Japanese and French, and wrote Chinese characters. Though his vision was not good, when he wasn't working he always carried a small Chinese dictionary in his hand. 'Why,' I asked, 'do you always carry the little book?' He replied, 'I want to give an example to our younger inmates. I want them to continue to learn.' Thanks to my meeting with this priest and friends who knew about Buddhism, I learned about my religion."

At the end of 1979 the prisoners were moved to a third camp, where they would remain for the next eight years. "If we stayed in any one place for a long time, we might create connections or try to escape," Nguyen explains. "When you are in the camp they move you around, change your work groups, shuffle you like a deck of cards, move you from room to room so you are not in a position to know your friends. They wanted to keep us disorganized. . . .

"Before taking you to another room they checked your belongings. When we were in our first camp I did not have anything. But later on I had letters from my family and items that were very precious and personal. So you have things you have to hide. This made it very tense. We did everything possible to keep those secret things safe because if they found them we would be punished severely. Usually it was confinement. They would shut you up in total isolation and darkness for weeks. One friend who had received this punishment told me, 'I called out my name lest I forget my own name. Sometimes you feel that your soul has dissolved.'"

Among Nguyen's cache of precious items were poems and letters he wrote to his wife on pieces of tissue-thin paper measuring barely 6 by 10 inches. The minuscule writing covered both sides of the paper, edge to edge. "I wrote every day, a tiny bit, because if one spent too much time writing, people would notice," he recalls. "One letter took about two weeks. I had a little tin box that had contained medication. I put all these letters in the box and buried the box in the garden. When I was moved from room to room in the same camp, I dug it up."

The residential area of the camp was a huge building divided into about ten rooms. "There were from 100 to 220 men in a room," Nguyen says. "There was an aisle in the middle and on both sides were elevations where people slept. You had to climb a ladder to reach the higher levels. Our living space for each person was less than one meter wide. Sometimes the space was so tight you slept on your side.

"In jail I did many things for my captors. I grew rice and vegetables, worked building houses, and worked in a quarry. We had a chisel and a piece of dynamite. I held the chisel at arm's length while younger, stronger men hit the chisel. When they hit the chisel it vibrated all the way through my chest to my heart. Then we put dynamite in the hole. I jumped into pools of lime with water and sand to make mortar for plaster.

"They picked young men to head up the work groups. Because he was being bribed, our work group leader was eager to help them [the guards] and he used to drive us harder. After work, when all we wanted to do was sleep, he forced us to sit up and he pointed to people who had not done as good a job as others because they were old or sick. . . . One day I was in his group when he got hurt. At that time I was in the infirmary with him. There was nobody there except us. He asked me, 'Do you think we can get out of here one day?' I told him, 'You are young. You will get out. I am sure of it. But that is not important. What is important is what you will be when you get out. Before coming in you had defects. This time in jail you have become more arrogant and cruel than you were before. If you try to correct yourself in jail and try to be better, then when you get out you will not have wasted your time. In fact, your time will have been properly spent.'" The young man did not say a word, but he listened.

The biggest event that occurred in the later years of Nguyen's imprisonment was the prisoners' acquisition of a radio. A guard asked Nguyen's work group if anyone knew how to fix his broken radio. A prisoner repaired it and that night listened to Voice of America and the BBC. The inmates bought the radio for gold from the guard, and for a year it supplied them news of the outside world. The appointed guardian of the radio, a former major with exceptional recall, listened to the radio at night, memorizing the songs and the news. The next day a designated man from each of the ten rooms of the camp listened to the major's account and then told the others. Since the men did not recognize many of the names in the news, they asked Nguyen to explain the news and put it in a proper context. "The radio helped our morale a great deal," he says. "It gave us hope."

It also entertained them with popular American songs. "Before, in my life outside, I had never listened to music," Nguyen says. "In Vietnam music had been used for propaganda, to shout slogans. But this music was about beauty and love and human passions. We sang ballads—'Three Coins in the Fountain,' 'Lara's Song' from *Dr. Zhivago,* and [the theme from] *The Bridge over the River Kwai.* This became our music and we sang it to defy our captors. When the young cadres [guards] heard this music, they asked us to teach them these songs."

Nguyen and his exhausted work party were trudging back to the camp one day when they heard one of their favorite songs being sung. At first it was faint and far away, then it grew louder. Looking up they saw a guard on the branch of a tree, singing.

The year of the radio ended when an informant reported its existence to the prison administration. The radio's guardian was taken away; a few days later the prisoners learned that he had been beaten to death. The identity of the informant did not remain unknown to the prisoners for long. One prisoner slept in the bathroom all night, waiting for the informant to come in so he could kill him, but his fellow prisoners pleaded with Nguyen to stop him because the reprisals would be far worse. "I talked to him for one hour," he says. "He did not say a word, just listened to me. But he did not kill the informer."

Nguyen suspects that the North Vietnamese, over time, came to believe that sending political prisoners to the North was a mistake. By the mid-1980s, thanks to international pressure, camp restrictions began to relax. Prisoners began to receive supplies and money from their families. The cadres began to treat the prisoners more humanely. Some cadres told wives of the prisoners that they could bring money to their husbands without registering it with the camp administration, a rule that once had been strictly enforced. "We trusted them, and my wife gave a large sum to a cadre," Nguyen says. "That night there was a tap on my window and the cadre gave me the money. I tried to give him a reward, but he refused. 'This is your money from your wife,' he said. 'Your wife spent so much money to come here.'"

On their way to and from work, prisoners filed past a checkpoint where the cadre in charge counted them and checked the possessions they had with them. One day the checkpoint supervisor, an important official whose daughter had married an officer, asked one of the prisoners, the former chief of a Saigon hospital, for help for his sick wife. The prisoner referred the cadre to a Dr. Que, a prisoner whose wife sent him medical supplies from their home in France. After hearing the symptoms, Dr. Que gave the cadre the supplies for several injections for his ailing wife.

When she recovered, the cadre's attitude toward the prisoners changed. Somehow the guards didn't discover outgoing letters from inmates that prisoners concealed in their clothes before going to see their wives. When Nguyen's wife came to visit, she slipped him a packet of letters for the inmates. When he passed his checkpoint, a cadre felt the letters inside his shirt, but Nguyen had only to say, "They are for Dr. Que," to be passed through.

This change in the attitudes of the guards made a powerful impression on Nguyen. Some cadres would approach him after work and ask to talk with him. Others gave him and his fellow prisoners food, despite the guards' own poverty.

Freedom, of a Sort
By the fall of 1987, Nguyen knew that the United States, through General John Vessey of Minnesota, was negotiating for the release of South Vietnam's remaining political prisoners. About ten o'clock one morning, Nguyen's work group heard an unexpected sound: the gong that usually signaled the beginning and end of their work shifts. The cadres guarding them in the field said the

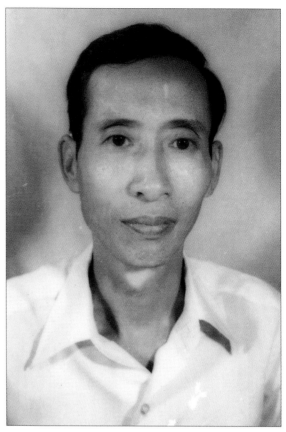

Diem Ngoc Nguyen in Saigon immediately following his release from a Communist concentration camp in 1987. The photograph was required for his identity card.

prisoners had to return to the camp, that the ringing of the gong at this unusual hour might signal something important. When they arrived, the prison administrator told them that they were being released. Nguyen's twelve-year imprisonment was over. Later that day, with cameras from Eastern Europe television stations rolling, the prisoners were loaded into cars that would take them to the train station. The long road from the camp to the entrance gate was lined with cadres and their wives and children, all waving and crying.

The captain of the camp and the cadre whose wife had been cured by Dr. Que accompanied the prisoners from the camp to the station where they were to catch the train for South Vietnam. "You would think these two men would be some kind of hardened Communists," Nguyen says. "But they stood there and waved and waved until our train was quite out of their sight.

"In the prison camp I saw hearts that became mellow and humane. That is why I do not have any hate or antipathy toward these people. All of them are victims of this terrible regime and ideology. If I still have some resentment and hatred, it is for the regime and ideology, and not for these poor people."

The trip to the South took four days. When word spread that railcars of released political prisoners were attached to the train, other passengers brought them food. When the train stopped in a large town, two boys came to its windows to sell ice cream. Nguyen and his one-time inmates had not seen ice cream for twelve years. When they eagerly offered their money, the boys refused to take it, saying, "No, our parents said that if we see uncles who are going south, the ice cream is free. Do not take money." Nguyen noticed that the boys were shivering in their thin shirts in the chill September air. He and his friends took off their heavy quilted cotton coats and handed them through the window to the boys.

When they arrived in Saigon, the former prisoners were loaded back onto buses and taken to a local prison. After a brief speech and distribution of documents, officials led the prisoners out of the building in a long, thin line. Waiting in the crowd for Nguyen were his wife, his twenty-two-year-old son, and his twenty-three-year-old daughter. Nguyen got on the back of his son's bicycle and the young man peddled his father, the diplomat, home. Nguyen weighed eighty-five pounds.

Nguyen and his wife talked late into the night. The next morning, when he went to the police station to get his papers, he learned that he would not be allowed to live with his wife and children unless he were registered and certified as dwelling in their apartment. He soon realized that he had simply exchanged one prison for a much larger one. Although life after imprisonment was far better, Nguyen was never free from fear. At least once a week, often in the middle of the night, an official in charge of neighborhood security would pound on their door and ask to see who was in the house. "They checked to make sure all four of us were there," Nguyen says. "If we had had an additional person, they would have asked, 'Who are you? What are you doing here?' And they would ask my wife, who at that time was the head of the household, 'Why is he here?' Or if I were missing, they would want to know where I was. You had to explain and explain."

From time to time a police officer from Hanoi came to Saigon to question Nguyen. The officer would offer to get him a job, but Nguyen always turned it down. "You never wanted to owe them anything," he explains. "I told them I gave private lessons in English and French and received money from my mother in the States." (Nguyen's mother and his five siblings were already living in the United States.)

Despite the hazard to themselves, many friends with whom he had been close—former students, teachers, and friends from the camp—came to visit Nguyen. "They came to see me right away, in spite of everything, because they understood," he recalls. "But other people were so afraid that they could not come to see me. I understood that as well." Both he and his visitors had to be careful. If a police officer were questioning him in his apartment, his son would stand guard on the first floor and deflect any friends who stopped by.

From time to time, Nguyen was ordered to report to police headquarters and inform them of his activities, naming the visitors he had had and what they had talked about. When he returned home, he would ask his wife and children to go tell his friends, "Today Nguyen was asked to report to the police and he did not mention you in his report. So please do not say anything about it." When his friends were then questioned by the police, they were always able to tell the same story.

A large tourist hotel in Saigon carried *Time* and *Newsweek* in English, magazines that were more expensive than Nguyen could afford. Nevertheless, almost every week, he or one of his friends would slip into the hotel, buy a copy, hide it in his shirt, and take it home, where it would be passed around to eager readers. At night they listened to Voice of America and the BBC on the radio.

The legislation signed between Washington and Hanoi that freed Nguyen from the prison camp also provided for the prisoners' resettlement in the United States via an organization called Humanitarian Operation. Although the legislation was signed in 1987 by North Vietnam's foreign minister and U.S. General John Vessey, it took two years for it to be implemented and almost four years before Nguyen's name appeared on an official resettlement list. When it did, he, his wife, and two grown children were given permission to leave South Vietnam. Each was allowed to bring forty-four pounds of luggage. Among Nguyen's possessions was the precious two-inch-thick packet of letters and poems he had written in prison and hidden so many times in the prison garden.

Coming to America

On March 8, 1991, when Nguyen and his family arrived in Washington, D.C., he was surprised and touched to be met at the airport by friends and members of the diplomatic corps who had worked with him in his overseas posts. For a week he was caught up in nonstop political discussions. The phone at his brother-in-law's home, where they were staying, rang continuously until late at night.

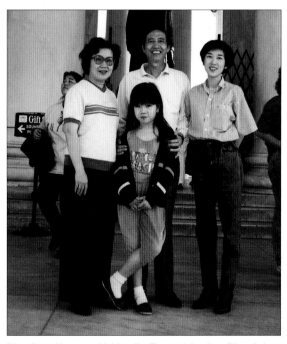

Diem Ngoc Nguyen with his wife, Thu, and daughter Diem Anh (at right) in front of the Jefferson Memorial in Washington, D.C., on March 10, 1991, two days after their arrival in the United States. The child is a niece, the daughter of Thu's brother.

After a week, Nguyen knew that if they stayed in Washington, he would once again become so engulfed in political life that he would not have enough time for his family. "I used to tell my wife, 'I work on a stage and act my part.' Now it was time for me to be a spectator and not act anymore. . . . I always remembered the time in 1979 when my wife and children came from Saigon to see me. They had had to ride for three days and four nights on a train and then rode from Hanoi on a truck loaded with coal. Their clothes were dirty and we had only fifteen minutes to see each other. So now I wanted to spend time with my family.

"It is why my wife and I wake up very early. We sit on the couch in the living room and have our coffee and talk about so many things. Or we don't have to talk about anything, but just sit there and enjoy each other's presence. It is a way to compensate for the time we lost."

Nguyen and his family immediately applied for U.S. citizenship. His mother, who was born in 1915, had already taken her citizenship examination in English. "We were all very proud when we took our oath," Nguyen says. "For me to become a U.S. citizen, to become American, does not mean I am less Vietnamese. I am a Vietnamese American. I have my Vietnamese values and now I apply American values as well. I feel much richer and very happy. . . .

"I am now free from fear. Fear is this kind of physical thing. It is in your viscera, in your intestines and your stomach. In the prison we had to show that we were not afraid. So we were very tense. When you are fearful, you have abdominal pain and diarrhea. When I came here, I thought having constipation and then diarrhea was my own physical problem. I told this to the psychologist and he said, no, emotion can affect your digestion.

"Perhaps it is only people like me who can appreciate this freedom from fear. Since I have been here, nobody has asked to see my papers. Nobody asks me who I am and who is with me in my house. When I go to buy a plane ticket, I just show my ID and that is it. When I go to Canada, I just show my passport and I can go. I don't talk about freedom as some kind of lofty ideal. Instead, when you are free from fear, you enjoy this in your body. . . . For me, this is the most precious thing, this freedom from fear."

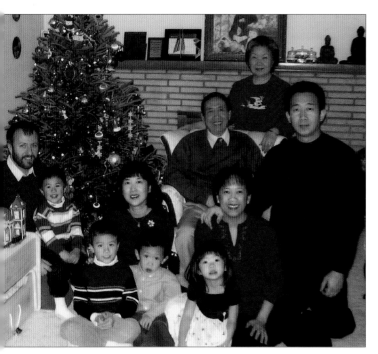

Diem and Thu Nguyen celebrate Christmas with their family in St. Paul in 2005. On the right is their son, Giao, with his wife, Mai Tram, and their two children, Jasmine Giao Chau and Giao Long. On the left is Diem's son-in-law, Jacques Gavois, and daughter, Diem Anh, and their sons, Rhone and Pyrenees.

When Nguyen and his family moved to St. Paul, Minnesota, they had little money and applied for food stamps and Medicaid. The experience was a positive one. "When we went to the office to ask for help, they treated us like people. We were not made to feel like we were beggars, humble or humiliated. They treated us so well." When Nguyen applied for housing, he was told that the waiting list for his preferred location was long, "but when we started to talk and when they learned that I had spent many years in jail, the interviewer told us that displaced persons should have a higher priority. . . . Two weeks later, she called and our house was ready. This human relationship we felt so much." When Nguyen's son bought a house, his parents moved in.

Driven by a desire to once again be of service, Nguyen applied for and landed the job as an interpreter at St. Paul–Ramsey Medical Center in 1994. He explains his happiness at getting the job by telling the story of a friend, another political prisoner who resettled in Boston. "My friend slept next to me in the camp for eight years," Nguyen recalls. "He had taught philosophy and sociology at the University in Saigon and had also been the vice minister of defense, a very important position. He spent longer than I did in prison and was not released until February of 1988. One day he called me from Boston, all excited about having landed a job as a storehouse watchman for the salary of eight dollars an hour. I told him that I shared his joy.

"For people like us, when we came to this country, we felt tired in our bones. When we were in jail, we had always talked of our families. I could not help my family while I was in jail. Instead I was a burden to them. Because of me, my children could not have a proper education, my family could not get a job. They were pariahs because of me. So we prisoners felt very responsible. When my friend talked about his thrill at getting a job at $8 an hour, I understood him perfectly. That is why, when I was offered this job at the hospital, I too was overjoyed. I was still of some use. I could help the Vietnamese patients and also repay my family."

In November 1997, three years after he was hired at St. Paul–Ramsey's International Clinic, Nguyen was given a signal honor: the President's Award. It read, "In recognition of outstanding performance serving the members and staff of Health Partners."

In 2005, the day after he retired, Nguyen at last took his dream trip to Paris.

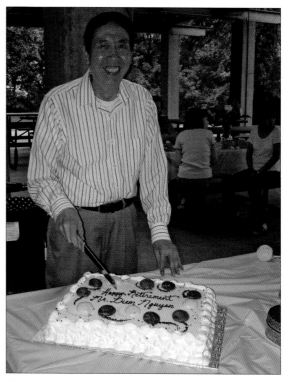

Diem Nguyen at his retirement party.

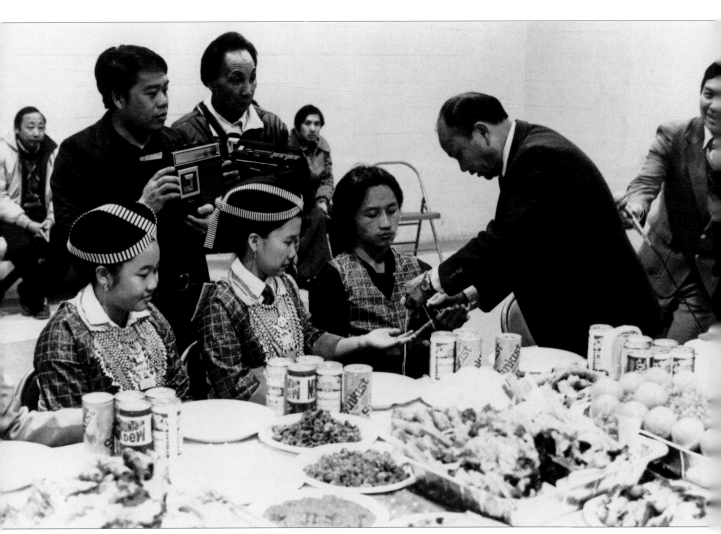

The revered Hmong general Vang Pao is asked for his blessing at a Hmong wedding reception in St. Paul in 1981. This is known as the baci ceremomy.

10: the Center for International Health

WHEN DR. NEAL HOLTAN founded the International Clinic in 1980, he was determined that it not become known as a place that helped only Southeast Asians, but all non–English-speaking people. Although the majority of his patients in the beginning were Hmong, Vietnamese, and Cambodian, that changed a decade later when events on the other side of the world brought a new kind of client—and a renewed sense of purpose—to the clinic.

In 1990, Russian president Boris Yeltsin declared his republic's economic sovereignty from the Soviet Union. While the Kremlin was reeling from this blow, elections in Estonia, Latvia, and Lithuania gave overwhelming victories to political parties that also favored independence. The Soviet Union was breaking up, and in the resulting turmoil, anti-Semitism—which had always been present in the USSR—became even more pronounced. Thousands of Soviet Jews sought asylum in the United States. Many settled in the Twin Cities, including Mikhail Perelman.

When Perelman came to America in late 1989, leaving his home and career in Samara, Russia, all the thirty-four-year-old could say in English was, "My name is Mikhail Perelman. I don't speak English." Eighteen years later, when asked why he left his country with only his wife, his twelve-year-old daughter, and two suitcases

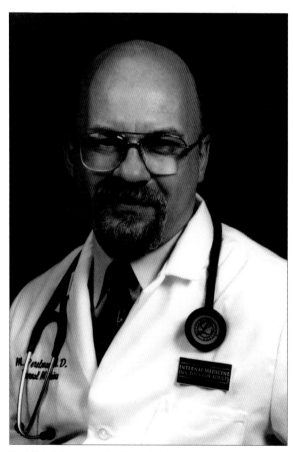

Dr. Mikhail Perelman, the Soviet Union physician who arrived in the United States speaking only Russian. He tackled medical texts in English with a dictionary, translating one page a day.

each, he replies, "I came here because of my last name."

To do anything in Russia, Perelman explains, you have to show your passport, which lists not only your name and address but also your nationality. His passport gave his nationality as Jewish, even though his Russian roots reach back untold generations. "I was Russian, but I had this stamp in my passport that said I was something else," he says. "I was not a religious Jew. In my city of one and a half million people, there was no synagogue. My parents were not religious. We had no symbols in our home. I think my grandparents from my father's side were religious, but they were killed in the Ukraine during the Second World War." It made no difference. Anti-Semitism was not written into Russian law, but it was embedded in practice.

"Everybody knew whom to blame for everything," Perelman says. "If there was no meat or clothes in the store, no running water, they knew whom to blame. When Gorbachev came, we felt relieved. Everything was open and it was much better. Then the government started to collapse and the people again blamed the Jews.

"Even before the Revolution there were pogroms. A Jew could not settle in the big cities; my great-grandparents could not live in St. Petersburg or Moscow. They had to live in the small villages that were appointed to them. That is why there were Jews leading the Revolution. Now the Russians blame the Jews for the Revolution too. 'It's your fault,' they say. 'You killed the Czars. It was much better before.'"

In Russia, his family was accomplished—his mother was a pediatrician, his brother a surgeon, Perelman himself an internist—but they felt like second-class citizens. When he applied for a fellowship in the department of health, one of his friends, whose mother Perelman had treated as a patient, asked him to withdraw his application. Word had come down from their superiors to select ten people for the fellowships, but no Jews. "Mikhail, I don't want you to be disappointed," his friend pleaded with him. "I don't want you to apply for this position because you will never be accepted."

The decision to immigrate to the United States was a difficult one for Perelman and his wife, Galina. At first they could not tell anyone their plans. Only after they had made an official request to depart could they talk openly about their decision. "We came [to the United States] at the end of 1989," he says. "People who came in the 1970s were very brave. They were called enemies of the people and traitors because they were leaving the Soviet Union. It was a terrible time. When I left, all my friends came to the airport to tell me goodbye. In the 1970s they would never have come."

"The Russians Are Coming"
Seemingly overnight, the usual mix of Cambodian, Vietnamese, and Hmong patients waiting in the narrow hallway of the International Clinic included the Twin Cities' newest immigrants: hundreds of middle-aged, professionally trained Russians. Upon the newcomers' arrival, Jewish Family Services of Minneapolis directed them to the clinic for medical care. Director Pat Walker

was thrilled. "Even though most of our patients had brown skins and the Russians had white," she recalls, "Jewish Family Services realized that, because of our cross-cultural competence, our clinic was the right place for them."

Walker quickly discovered that the clinic's Russian patients were very good at working the system. If they could get a letter from their physician certifying that they were diabetic or had high blood pressure, for instance, they could get more food stamps. A letter from a doctor explaining that one partner of a couple had a medical condition requiring therapeutic equipment to be used at night could get them a two-bedroom apartment in subsidized housing. Soon Walker and her staff were swamped with requests for letters that justified applications for government assistance with housing and health care. "If the social system structure were better, our doctors wouldn't have to do that," she laments. "Doctors in other clinics don't like to write letters. It is too much work, the patients' needs are too complicated, and there are too many demands that are not medical issues." Many petitioners did not see why such letters could not be provided instantly in the middle of a busy clinic day. After a few months, Walker had to establish ground rules: the clinic would produce the letters but had a week in which to do so.

Working the system also meant that the Russian immigrants insisted on being seen by specialists for common ailments that the clinic's internists could easily treat. If a Russian patient came in for a skin-tag removal, for example, he would demand to see a dermatologist. Someone with a stomach problem would announce, "I must see the gastroenterologist." A perplexed Walker called Jewish Family Services for advice on interpreting the phenomenon. The resettlement expert replied, "Just send me the doctors' resumes."

Because the Russian patients at the International Clinic were on Medicaid and Medicare, they assumed that St. Paul–Ramsey was a public hospital that served only the poor. In the Soviet Union's two-tiered medical system, the public hospital cost little or nothing but the care was substandard and only the worst of doctors practiced there. Private clinics cost more but offered the best care and they were staffed with specialists. Once they saw the prestigious institutions where the physicians had studied and trained, the Russian patients' skepticism changed to pride. "Did you see that my doctor, Dr. Walker, studied at Mayo?" they bragged to each other.

Despite the initial additional burdens placed on her staff, Walker sympathized with her Russian patients. Perseverance was how they had survived in Russia, where they had stood for hours in long lines for items as basic as bread. These older professionals—engineers, scientists, physicians—were now living on fixed incomes. Because they could no longer work in their professions, they had lost their sense of identity. An extra $65 worth of food stamps represented a major improvement in their lives and self-esteem.

"When I come here I could not work in my profession," says Estra, a fifty-eight-year-old Russian whose rheumatoid arthritis is treated by Walker at the clinic. "I was a builder, a draftsman." Estra is weary after taking three buses to the clinic from her home in Apple Valley. She slumps in her chair in an examining room and shakes her head. "I know I need go finish college. My English not good. I take two-year course to be teacher assistant. I like work in a school. Very good environment. Children like me. I feel better when I work with children."

Though she suffers from arthritis, Estra's major complaint is depression. She has four children, none of whom are well. Until recently, she taught art and craft projects and supervised the lunchroom at a small private school in her neighborhood. When the school downsized, she wasn't rehired. She thinks she may have been discriminated against because she is not an American.

Walker talks to Estra about her depression and asks her to try to find something to be happy about every day—to find five minutes of joy. Estra listens carefully but replies, "I'm not positive in my heart."

Cardiac Mystery

Other heart problems involving her older Russian immigrants began to profoundly concern Walker. Every week, seemingly without fail, the clinic would admit a Russian patient, sixty or older, with some kind of cardiovascular emergency—atrial fibrillation, acute chest pain, heart attacks, strokes. Time after time Walker would need only a quick look at a patient in distress before deciding to start him on nitroglycerin, oxygen, and IVs while having someone call for a gurney to transport him to the cardiac ICU. In the Health Center for Women, where she worked simultaneously with patients the same age as the

Russians, Walker might see two incidents a year of the sort that were occurring weekly in the International Clinic. What was going on?

The more she thought about the Russians' cardiac problems, the more Walker realized that she and her staff were going at the problem backward. "We should be on the other end of this," she said. Research revealed that a Russian diet of fatty foods was the culprit: bread spread with a thick layer of lard, regular consumption of soured buttermilk called kefir, and a lot of potatoes. Walker tried to imagine what it must be like for Russian immigrants, coming from a society of scarcity, to walk into an American grocery store and confront fifty kinds of breakfast cereal. "They didn't know how to read the labels, so they bought the sugar-frosted flakes because they tasted good," she says.

The solution was to do something to prevent (or at least ameliorate) the heart problems before they became acute. Walker decided to organize an education program for the Russian immigrants at the St. Paul Jewish Community Center. To fund it she applied for a grant from the Jay and Rose Phillips Family Foundation, the family that had established Mount Sinai Hospital, whose emergency room Walker had once run. It was a perfect match—Jay and Rose Phillips were the children of Russian Jewish immigrants, Rose Phillips had heart disease—and Walker got the grant. When she received a second grant to hire a Russian interpreter, Basil Ivanov, for a year, the heart-health education program was launched in 1999. When the grant money ran out for Ivanov, Walker appealed to hospital CEO Jim Dixon. "It looks like the Russians are coming," he remarked, and took over the funding for the interpreter.

For two hours every Wednesday for ten weeks, the Russian immigrants who attended the program learned relaxation techniques, age-appropriate exercises, and, most popular of all, lectures on the heart and nutrition. Every session was filled and there was a long waiting list. Each ten-week session ended with a celebration, the presentation of certificates of completion, and a dinner of heart-healthy dishes prepared by the Russian participants. Walker was amazed to learn that all of her Russian patients had blood pressure cuffs in their homes and took their blood pressure daily. One man, an engineer, made a graph charting the mean of his blood pressure over a month. Significantly, the number of Russians coming to the clinic with heart ailments began to drop as patients read their nutrition labels, walked daily, and took their medications for high cholesterol and diabetes.

Walker knew she had hit a home run with her education program when one of her Russian patients, a woman she had been treating for a cardiac condition, came in for her appointment. When Walker asked her about her chest pain, the woman beamed and replied, "My darling Patricia! My heart it is *delicious!*" Other Russian patients wrote notes of appreciation to the clinic staff. Wrote one, "Everyone who knows you loves you because you are the best people I've known. You help people and God bless you." Another wrote, "You will always swim in the ocean of love." One patient brought cans of beans and boxes of cheese, commodities she had been given, to share with the nurses.

Overextended as usual, Walker nonetheless taught the anatomy section of the heart-health program for its first year. She then asked a Russian doctor from Minneapolis to take her place. That doctor was Mikhail Perelman, who had at last reestablished his medical career a decade after immigrating to America.

Upon their arrival in the United States, Perelman's daughter, Jenny, who had completed the sixth grade in Russia, was placed in the ninth grade in her Minneapolis public school. (She later skipped twelfth grade and went directly to the University of Minnesota.) Her father found it harder going. No one would hire him. After a year he finally found a job as a home health aide, washing and shaving clients and preparing their meals.

After spending three weeks in an English class, he began reading English-language textbooks at the University of Minnesota medical library. "I had a dictionary beside me and I could read only one page a day," he recalls. He then began taking the medical examinations he had passed long ago in Russia—anatomy, physiology, biochemistry—this time in English. The charge for each exam was $500, a large sum for his struggling family.

Perelman took the first examination and did not pass. He took the second exam and failed that one as well. "I didn't pass because I could not understand the questions, not because I was stupid," he explains. "I did not know the words, what they were asking me. You cannot bring a dictionary to the examinations, only a pencil." On the third try he passed his first exam. It was 1992, three years after he had arrived in the United States.

When he passed the internal medicine and surgery exams, as well as a difficult English language proficiency test, Perelman began looking for a hospital where he could take his residency. "I could not find a residency here in the Twin Cities," he says. "Nobody wanted to accept me. They told me I was too old. I was thirty-seven." Eventually, he was offered residencies in family practice in New York and in internal medicine in Detroit. With his daughter and wife settled in school and at work in the Twin Cities, Perelman spent three years at Detroit's Wayne State University to complete his training.

On Perelman's first day of residency, a doctor sent him to do blood work on a patient, adding almost as an afterthought, "This is an HIV patient, so be careful." Perelman had never seen an HIV patient in Russia. In the Soviet Union he had dealt with problems of alcohol abuse, but in Detroit the problems were drugs and violence. "When we worked in urgent care, it was like being in a war zone," he remembers. "People had gunshot wounds, knife wounds—it was terrible. People told me not to go out of the hospital after dark. 'Sleep here, but don't go outside. It is dangerous.' Detroit was not a nice place to work, but I was happy to have found a residency. During my residency I passed the last of my examinations and the board exam." It had taken him ten years to get back to where he had been professionally when he left the Soviet Union.

"If someone were to ask me, right now, would you recommend [immigration], I would tell him to think about it, because it is very tough," Perelman says. He knows he's one of the lucky ones. He knows other Russian physicians in the United States who are selling cars or working in stores because they could not pass their examinations.

Perelman was back in the Twin Cities and working in a Minneapolis clinic when Pat Walker brought him to St. Paul to work in her cardiac education program at the Jewish Community Center. She wanted him to join her staff at the International Clinic, but she could not invite him to do that until major organizational changes took place at St. Paul–Ramsey Medical Center.

Cross-Cultural Care

While it had been Neal Holtan's goal for the International Clinic to serve patients from all non–English-speaking cultures, both he and Pat Walker also envisioned it to be multidisciplinary, representing many medical specialties working together. They had not been able to bring this about successfully because of the way medicine was administratively organized at St. Paul–Ramsey. Each department within the medical center's clinics—internal medicine, pediatrics, obstetrics and gynecology, psychiatry, psychology—worked in its own administrative "silo," with little incentive to cooperate with one another. When physicians did cooperate, they crossed departmental and budgetary lines, which further complicated their efforts.

Things began changing in 1993, when St. Paul–Ramsey Medical Center merged with Health Partners, a Twin Cities–based health maintenance organization. In 1996 the Ramsey Clinic physicians formed the Health Partners Medical Group, and in 1997 Health Partners bought St. Paul–Ramsey Medical Center and renamed it Regions Hospital. Physicians who were not comfortable working outside a departmental structure left; others who liked the multidisciplinary approach to medicine stayed. In the resulting shuffle, Walker saw an opportunity for the International Clinic to become the Center for International Health—to reach its potential as a multidisciplinary service offering cross-cultural care.

In her carefully prepared presentation to the Health Partners Care Delivery Leadership Team, Walker explained that she wanted more than a new name for the clinic. She wanted "to provide high-quality, culturally competent care, enhanced through professional education and research, to our community of refugees and immigrants." She also wanted a separate budget so she could hire her own physicians, psychologists, nurses, and physicians' assistants to create a staff that looked like and spoke the languages of her patients.

When the leadership team gave its approval, it meant that Walker had her own organization to run, with the authority to hire and fire, to spend money as she saw fit, and to organize the clinic to more effectively provide health care across the boundaries of race and culture. "I had a budget I could control and spend the way I wanted to," she remembers. "That was when we could tighten things up. I thought a lot about what we were trying to do here and how to create the best care-delivery model."

A critical first step for Walker in forming the new Center for International Health was to find the right nurse manager, one who was assigned full-time to the clinic and one who had experience working overseas. Walker's younger sister, Elizabeth Anderson, and

their old American Refugee Committee connections came to the rescue when they crossed paths again with public health nurse Bridget Votel. Votel had worked for ARC all over Africa, first running a feeding program for 140,000 refugees in the Sudan, then working in Kenya, Rwanda, Tanzania, and Malawi. In 1998, when Votel was back in the Twin Cities, Walker offered her the nurse-manager job.

"I had been profoundly changed by my refugee experience," Votel says. "It affected every part of my work. I was attracted to the Center for International Health because these were health-care professionals I could relate to. We shared a mission and had a similar philosophy of service." She and Walker wanted to ensure that the support staff and provider staff were a mirror of the communities that they served. They wanted the center's health workers to speak the same language or to have the same cultural experiences as their patients. One of their first hires was Mikhail Perelman.

"Visitors to our clinic often say, 'You know, the atmosphere in your clinic is unusual,'" Perelman says. "It is not like in other American clinics. Everybody here wants to help each other.

"We know how our patients feel, what they are going though, because we had the same experience," he adds. "Right now, I have a lot of Russian patients. They come to me not only because I speak Russian, which is a big deal for them because they can express themselves without an interpreter, but because they know that I had the same experience when I came to this

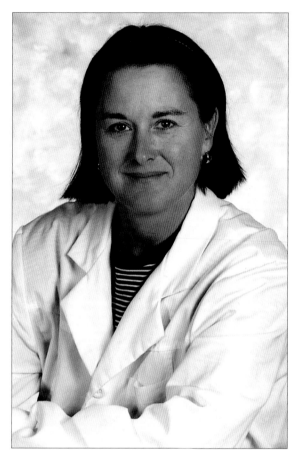

Public health nurse Bridget Votel's experience in refugee camps in many countries was invaluable in developing the cross-cultural program at the Center for International Health.

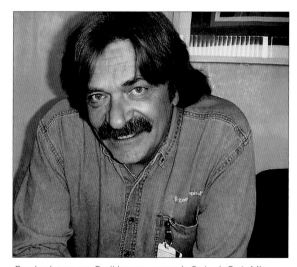

Russian interpreter Basil Ivanov grew up in St. Louis Park, Minnesota, where he learned Russian from his immigrant parents.

country. I know what they are going through. . . . I can understand them better than the traditional American doctor who went from high school to college to medical school and did not experience anything else in his life."

"The key [to cross-cultural care]," adds Walker, "is attitudes, skills, and knowledge." Health practitioners in the United States must have attitudes toward their patients that are neither racist nor patronizing and that do not stereotype people. If American doctors do not speak the language of their immigrant patients, they must make use of professional interpreters. If they don't know a patient's culture, they must learn it. And American doctors must be aware of and be able to recognize the diseases that their patients from other lands are likely to have, whether they're immigrants or long-term visitors.

American doctors need to know, for instance, that they should routinely screen a Liberian patient for malaria, even if that person has no symptoms, because malaria is common in Liberia. That soldiers fighting in Iraq might be infected with leishmaniasis, a parasitic disease that is spread by sand flies and causes skin ulcers or, more seriously, attacks the liver and spleen and can prove fatal. That 85 percent of Asians are lactose-intolerant and avoid dairy products because they cause diarrhea, and so doctors should check for osteoporosis about ten years sooner in Asian women than in American women. That 19 percent of Vietnamese are carriers for hepatitis B and that Koreans have a greater than 15 percent chance of being a carrier, so they should be routinely screened for hepatitis.

The importance of routine screening hit home with Walker during her physical examination of a Korean woman who was adopted as an infant and had lived for thirty-two of her thirty-three years in the United States. Noting her patient's place of birth, Walker asked if she had ever been tested for hepatitis B, explaining that in less developed countries, 50 percent of hepatitis B is transmitted at birth from mother to baby. If she were a carrier, the woman had a 33 percent chance of developing cirrhosis of the liver or liver cancer. The woman had seen as many as ten physicians over her lifetime, yet none had ever asked whether she'd been tested for the disease.

The woman's test came back positive: she *was* a carrier. She now gets a blood test every six months for liver cancer and an ultrasound of her liver every year. "If you do frequent screens, you can find these cancers when they are small, take them out, and patients have a longer survival rate," Walker explains. "This young woman is prominent in the Korean adoptees network, and after her experience, she wrote an article about hepatitis B in the Korean community that went out over the Internet."

More sobering was the case of a fifty-one-year old Cambodian man who came to the clinic complaining of ringing in his ear. When Walker examined his face and neck, she detected an enlarged lymph node on his cheek in front of his ear. She sent him to an ear, nose, and throat surgeon, asking the specialist to screen the man for nasopharyngeal carcinoma since there is a high incidence of the cancer in China. "I don't think he has an enlarged lymph node," the surgeon reported back after examining the man's neck. "This is just regular old ringing in the ear. Don't worry about it."

Walker saw the patient four months later and again was sure she felt an enlarged lymph node. "I am really worried about this," she told the surgeon in referring the patient a second time. "Please do a CAT scan." The surgeon did the scan, which revealed that the man had advanced nasopharyngeal cancer. The patient died within a year. Walker was so upset that she has made certain that everyone in the Center for International Health knows that if they see an Asian patient with ringing in one ear, they are not to assume that the ringing is the result of ear damage from a bomb exploding nearby. While that is a possibility, doctors must also screen for cancer.

Building a Reputation

In 1997, Walker and her Center for International Health colleague, psychiatrist Jim Jaranson, published one of the first comprehensive medical journal articles in the United States on refugee and immigrant health. The article defined the field of immigrant health care and posed questions about and recommendations for providing that care: What kinds of screening should be done in a clinic serving refugees and immigrants? What are the common diseases of these populations? How should such clinics deal with parasites and tuberculosis?

After the article was published, Walker began getting calls from practitioners across the country who previously had felt isolated in their attempts to deal with immigrant patients. Their questions were varied:

"I've got some people with TB. How can I get them to take their medications?"

"What do we do about hookworm?"

"Can we use the same screening test on an African patient from Sierra Leone as we use on the Hmong?"

"Should an annual physical examination for a Vietnamese patient be different from the one we give our American patients?"

What quickly became clear was that health workers across the United States were dealing with issues they had rarely encountered in medical school and with situations that were preventing large populations from receiving adequate health care. Walker spent more and more of her time speaking on the topic throughout North America and consulting over the phone. Medical questions were mingled with systems questions: How was the Center for International Health financed? How did the hospital administration deal with the plight of refugees and immigrants?

"Cross-cultural care" was becoming the new catch phrase in medicine and Walker its best-known proponent. Since returning from Thailand in 1988, she had attended every national meeting she could on refugee and immigrant health, on tropical and travel medicine updates, and on disparities in immigrant health care. Her regional reputation in the field became wider spread as she spoke to various groups about refugee health concerns. By December 1998, when the *Journal of Ambulatory Care* invited her to publish a description of the cross-cultural care model she had developed at the Center

for International Health, Walker's national reputation was without question.

Even back at Mayo Medical School, where Walker had studied and trained, her influence was felt. On her way to catch a flight to New Orleans to give a lecture on cross-cultural care, she ran into her former professor of internal medicine and Mayo mentor, Dr. Henry Schultz. Schultz reminded her that she had been the first Mayo medical student to serve overseas. "We percolated along for about fifteen years after you left and didn't get very far," he admitted. "But once we offered the overseas experience at the level of graduate medical education, it really took off. Your trip to Thailand was the inspiration for setting up our international rotations for students and residents. We don't thank you on our Web site, but we should."

Communities around the country that were experiencing waves of immigrants—Seattle, Chicago, Boston, and others—regularly asked Walker to share her expertise and knowledge with their physicians. "Maine had this big influx of Cambodians from Boston, and Lewiston experienced a huge migration of people from Somalia," she explains. "It made the national news and my name just floated to the top."

The Twin Cities also were seeing an increase in Somali immigrants—a number that would eventually become the largest concentration of Somalis in the United States. Once again, just as the Russian immigrants had done a decade earlier, the Twin Cities' newest refugees were finding their way to the Center for International Health. Once again, Pat Walker began hiring more foreign-born staff, starting with Somali physician Fozia Abrar.

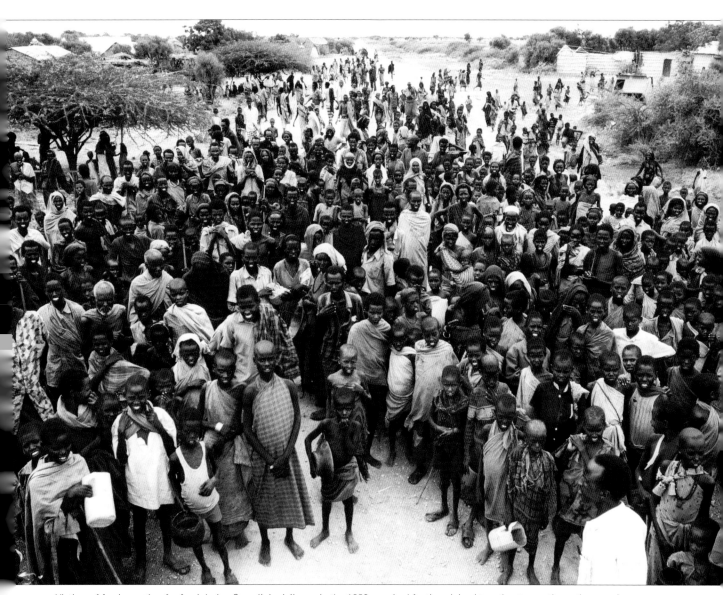

Victims of famine gather for food during Somalia's civil war. In the 1980s warlord factions joined together to overthrow then president Siad Barre, who finally lost power in 1991. Since then the civil war has consisted of power struggles between warlords, ravaging the country with famine.

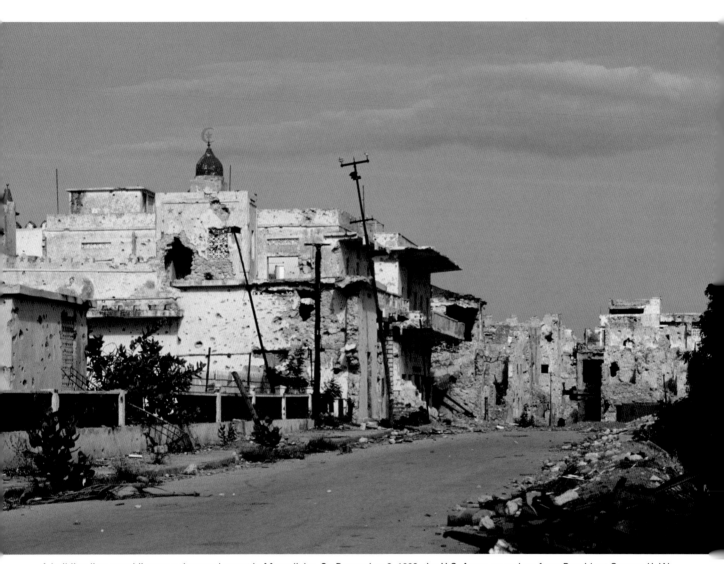

A building lies crumbling on a deserted street in Mogadishu. On December 3, 1992, the U.S. Army, on orders from President George H. W. Bush, launched Operation Restore Hope, both to protect relief workers whose jobs were becoming increasingly difficult due to clan violence in the city and to feed starving people following a prolonged drought.

11: an international staff

THE RESIDENCY DIRECTOR of the clinic next to the Center for International Health ran into Pat Walker one day and introduced her to a physician who was beginning her fellowship in occupational medicine at Regions Hospital. As they walked along, the new doctor mentioned that she was from Somalia. Walker came to an abrupt halt in the hospital corridor.

"You must come to work in my clinic!" she exclaimed. "We are seeing more and more patients from Somalia."

The physician was Fozia Abrar. The year was 2000, and the decade-long civil war in Somalia had driven thousands from their homes to whatever country would give them refuge, including the United States. Hundreds were arriving weekly in Minnesota.

Walker once again went to work on the hospital administration, and within a few days Abrar was assigned to divide her time between her fellowship responsibilities and caring for Somali patients at the Center for International Health. When Abrar's fellowship ended, she began working full-time in the center as the first Somali doctor on staff at Regions Hospital.

Dr. Fozia Abrar

Abrar's appointment to the Center for International Health after a chance meeting in a hospital corridor was only the latest in the series of extraordinary events that had marked her life and defined her career.

When Abrar was a child in Somalia, the East African country was divided into three colonial protectorates: British, French, and Italian. Abrar lived with her family in the British sector. As independence movements sprouted up across the globe in the wake of

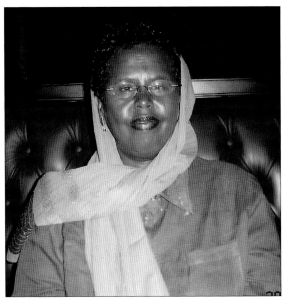

Dr. Fozia Abrar grew up in the British sector of Somalia.

World War II, colonial administrations began closing down. With Somalia's protectorate set to end in 1960, the British government attempted to train native Somalians to fill the official posts once held by colonial administrators. As part of this program, Abrar's father was sent first to a university in Belgium to become a public-health nurse and then to a university in London to study hygiene.

Although her father, Adam Abrar, had grown up illiterate, he had had the good fortune to work for a British public-health official who recognized Abrar's keen intelligence and taught him to read and write in English. After his studies abroad, Abrar returned to Somalia and became a deputy director in the Ministry of Public Health. Part of his responsibilities was the implementation of a program to eliminate smallpox worldwide. As a child, Fozia accompanied her father into Somalian villages, where she helped inoculate children against the disease. "That is where I became interested in public health," she says.

After working for five years on the smallpox program, Adam Abrar was hired by the World Health Organization and the family moved to Geneva, Switzerland. Other postings in Nigeria and Ghana followed. Fozia graduated from high school in Somalia, which was now being strongly influenced by the Soviet Union, and was studying to apply to medical school in Ghana when she received a scholarship to attend medical school in Hungary. Already fluent in English, French, and Somali, she also had to learn Hungarian and Latin, the languages in which her medical school courses were taught.

Disaster struck the family in 1982, when Fozia's father died in a plane crash in Somalia. He had always wanted his daughter to attend the Oxford School of Public Health and then return to work in Somalia. That plan died with her father. She had one year remaining in medical school, and when she graduated she returned to Somalia, where civil war was raging.

"The civil war in Somalia was a big shock," Fozia Abrar says. "People walked out of their homes with just the clothes they had on. If they carried anything, they were mobbed. They walked for days and days to safety. Many were middle-class. A small child asked my aunt why everything on the ground was red. My aunt replied that the red was paint; she could not bring herself to tell the child it was blood."

Refugees were massed on Somalia's western border with Ethiopia, and the Swedish Church Relief Organization, which was running a refugee camp, needed a doctor. The organization hired Abrar, the only physician for fourteen thousand destitute and desperate people. She was twenty-two years old. Having entered medical school right out of high school, she had not participated in a residency program. She knew she needed more expert help than she could offer, so her first action upon arriving in the camp was to send for traditional healers. "They were capable of doing a lot of things," she says. "They showed me how to set bones. I was new and had never dealt with trauma. They knew better than I how to deal with it. The year I spent in the camp was my medical residency."

Much as Steve Miles and the American Refugee Committee had discovered in

Thailand, Abrar quickly realized that education was key to sustaining the Somali refugee camp's mission. Women were dying in childbirth, so she taught the midwives sterilization techniques. Babies were dying from diarrhea, so she showed aides how to make oral hydrations. She also taught them how to treat malaria and malnutrition, how to give drugs for HIV infections, and how to vaccinate children against measles.

After a year at the refugee camp and another four working as a doctor in Djibouti, a country along the northwest border of Somalia, Abrar decided to come to the United States. She was tired of people saying to her, "Why do you want a career? Why don't you marry and have children? You are a woman and this is all you can do." She wanted to specialize, and when the opportunity came to earn a master's degree in public health from Boston University, she took it.

After her graduation in 1989, however, Abrar quickly discovered that she could not practice any kind of medicine in the United States without certification. She couldn't even work as a nurse's aide. She took a job on the night shift in a youth correctional institution in Washington, D.C., for six dollars an hour. ("The kids were white and looking at me," she says. "They were afraid to go to sleep.") When Washington's Department of Public Health discovered Abrar, they put her to work in a program helping families affected by AIDS.

It was during her six years with that program, and with the encouragement of her coworkers, that Abrar studied for and passed the U.S. medical license exam.

"The examination is torture," she says. "It covers everything. It took me three years to complete all of it. You study, you fail, you take it again. The exams were $600 for each sitting. The last one was about $1,000. But I did it. I passed." Residencies in Washington and Boston hospitals completed her training. Following the Boston residency, she accepted the fellowship at Regions Hospital, where she met Pat Walker.

Diverse Needs, Diverse Solutions

After hiring Fozia Abrar, Walker continued recruiting bilingual, bicultural health-care workers to treat the center's increasingly diverse patients. To her Somali and Kenyan staff she added more Hispanic, Vietnamese, Hmong, and Cambodian workers, plus a corps of social workers, like Kathy Lytle, who untangle problems that stand in the way of people getting help.

"When I hire a physician or physician's assistant who is a refugee or who has worked in refugee camps, there is an unspoken understanding," Walker says. "I know that I won't have to train that person in cross-cultural health care."

When Russian internist Mikhail Perelman started working at the Center for International Health, he was impressed that almost everyone there had some international experience. "I was in shock when I first saw Dr. Pat Walker, a blond American lady, speaking Thai," he says. "Even Rob Carlson, a physician's assistant, spent six months in the Sudan."

Yet Perelman, an immigrant himself, had his own cultural barriers to overcome. "When I came to this clinic, I had never had contact with Hmong people," he says. "I did not know that they existed. So when I came, I asked my Hmong nurses to tell me about their culture—where they came from, why they were here. . . . When my Hmong patients came to me for the first time, they were very closed." He purses his lips and puts his finger up to them. "They were not smiling. They did not talk. I asked about their problems. 'I have an ache.' Silence. 'Where do you have it?' They would not answer, but would point to their stomachs."

Perelman also had to learn Somalia's customs. "My first Somali patient was a woman about fifty years old," he says. "When I came into the examining room, I greeted her and held out my hand. The patient, upset, backed away, crossed her arms over her chest, and said to the Somali interpreter, 'No, I cannot do this.' Then the interpreter explained, 'You cannot shake hands with our women, because when she gives her hand to another man it means that she is giving herself to this man.'"

With time, Perelman and his foreign-born patients learned to understand each other. "Now [the Hmong] are so friendly with me," he says. "They are smiling. They call out when they see me in the corridor. 'Hello, Doctor!' they say. . . . Now, when I come into the room where this same Somali woman patient is waiting, she is the first to offer me her hand. This warms my heart."

Abrar points out that all of the immigrants and refugees seen at the Center for International Health have lost everything—their homes, their relatives, their neighbors, their culture, a way of life they understand. Their sense of loss is profound. When they see

that their caregiver is respectful, compassionate, and not rushed or in a hurry, then they respond.

That's particularly true with the center's Somali patients, to whom the Western mentality of time is foreign. Internist Mohamud Afgarshe, a native of Somalia who joined the Center for International Health in September 1992, explains the reality of working with Somalis. "The first fifteen minutes of the twenty-minute appointment with a Somali patient must be spent in greetings," he says. "I must say, 'Good day. How are you? How is your father? How is your mother? How are your children?'"

"Dr. Afgarshe's experience really is true," Walker says. "If you do not first establish the relationship, the trust, nothing will happen thereafter."

She recalls the case of Mohammad, a young man who for ten years had had the Madura foot fungus infection. The only treatment was amputation of his foot. With a wife and young children to support, he was apprehensive about what would happen to him if he had the surgery. But when Walker referred Mohammad to a surgeon, the specialist became frustrated with his patient's anxious and endless questions about the procedure. The surgeon finally told Mohammad, "I'm tired of you repeatedly coming back to my office to talk about your foot. When you are ready to have the surgery, come back to see me. In the meantime, don't waste my time talking about it."

"I don't want to see him again," Mohammad later told Walker. "He doesn't care about me. He told me to come back when I was ready for surgery. But I have a lot of questions." She called another surgeon friend and explained Mohammad's problem. "This young man is really afraid about surgery, fearful that he is going to lose mobility. I have been moving him closer and closer to accepting surgery, and I think he is getting there, but what he needs now is some tender attention."

The second surgeon immediately grasped the situation. "I can help him," he said. "I'll refer him to a foot specialist, who can explain feet to him, and have him meet with someone who has lost a foot." That patience and willingness to spend time with the patient paid off. Mohammad had the operation, and, as it turned out, the surgeon was able to save part of Mohammad's heel.

Becoming angry with *any* patient is unacceptable, says Walker, referring to the first surgeon's handling of Mohammad's anxiety, but it is especially so with immigrants who, she believes, are uniquely vulnerable. "One of the fundamental principles in cross-cultural care is that you must respect the patient, be patient-centered, which means you have to accept the fact that the patient's timeline might be different from your own. And you must establish trust. The way you establish trust is to show not just empathy, but respect. I think people can tell the difference between a physician who is merely behaving empathically—something taught in medical school—versus the physician who really cares about them."

But Walker also recognizes that it isn't easy for her colleagues to adequately care for, in twenty minutes, their immigrant patients who do not speak English. "That is really hard," she says. "We are told, organizationally, to see a patient every twenty minutes, and we cannot vary it for the person who doesn't speak English. I understand the providers' frustration with the systems within which they work."

Compounding the frustration is the fact that making and keeping a clinic appointment can be a difficult concept for Somalis to grasp. They are accustomed to visiting a clinic when they feel like it, not at a predetermined time, and they expect to have to wait to be seen, so the time at which they arrive isn't critical. Likewise, if public transportation doesn't serve their neighborhood, it is hard for them to keep appointments or show up on time, and so they don't. Somali patients are often late because they are waiting for someone to pick them up.

One of Abrar's greatest challenges with her Somali patients is knowing that most of their ailments are preventable. Back in Somalia, the concept of preventive medicine, of going to a hospital for screening tests such as a mammogram or a Pap smear, was unknown to them. Somalis went to a hospital only if they were very sick.

Even if they do believe in preventive health care, patients not reared with a belief in the Western model of medicine may not accept the germ theory of disease. Illnesses may be blamed on mystical causes such as evil spirits, spells put on one by an enemy, or just desserts for not having been kind to one's parents or having fulfilled other family obligations. It is in warding off evil spirits and being a good person that illness is thwarted, they believe.

"I x-ray a patient's lungs and tell her she has pneumonia," Abrar says. "The patient may reply, 'You can call it what you want, but I know what is wrong with me. I have been a bad person, gossiping about people, and that is why I am sick.'

"The culture is Muslim," Abrar points out. "Many people believe that things are meant to happen and one cannot do anything about it. They believe that even the day you will die is predetermined. I talk with my mother, who has diabetes, and explain to her that she has to test her blood, control the sugar and carbohydrates she eats. She replies, 'Keep quiet. You are not Allah.'"

Many Somali become diabetic when they come to the United States and adopt American lifestyles. "The diet here is terrible," Abrar says. "In Somalia they drank camel's milk and ate vegetables at two meals a day, breakfast and lunch, with no dinner. Portions were smaller than in the United States and they never ate snacks between meals. People ate together, and a plate of food that would serve two in the United States would be enough for seven or eight people there. Food is not abundant in Somalia as it is here. I have a friend who gained sixty pounds when she came, eating doughnuts, bagels, cream cheese— foods that were new and exciting."

Somalis also don't get enough exercise, Abrar says. "Here in Minnesota, the Somali live in isolated, high-rise buildings and seldom walk to work or shopping. When I was growing up no one had a car. We would walk five miles to school and another five miles back. Since there was no refrigeration, women walked to the market daily. That walking was good for them."

Educating immigrants about the benefits of nutrition and preventive health care presents a challenge at the Center for International Health. "We must always aim for best practices as best we can," Walker admits. "I know it is easier not to do that with someone who does not speak English. It is easier to say, 'Take this pill,' knowing that, with an immigrant or refugee, the questions will not come back at us as they do from Westerners: 'What is this pill? What are my options? What are the risks? What are the side effects?' So we have to be proactive as providers to immigrants. We have to teach people about the Western care delivery system. We have to say, 'Let me tell you about this medicine, why I am choosing it, why it is so important for you to take it every day.'"

Regardless of the challenges, Walker says, a doctor's fundamental duty is to put the patient first. "We have to respect patients and their choices," she explains. "If I have an older patient with degenerative arthritis in her knee, my goal might be to get her pain relief, have her knee replaced, put her on an exercise program to strengthen her heart. The patient's goal might be, 'I just want to be able to walk up the stairs without hurting.' The point is to meet the patients around their personal goals, not ours."

Dr. Karen Ta
Adjusting to the center's "best practices" philosophy of care took some effort on psy-

chiatrist Karen Ta's part. "I enjoy working [at the Center for International Health]," Ta says, "though it is stressful at times. When I first started, my expectations were a lot higher. I thought I could fix the problems. Now I realize that I cannot do that—that I can just be here for our patients, day by day."

Ta, a psychiatrist with the Center for International Health since 1995, was thirteen years old when South Vietnam fell. Her father was a pharmacist and an officer in the South Vietnamese army; he was interned in a reeducation camp for three years. Her mother, who was a math teacher, supported the family during that time. The Communist regime did not allow Ta and her brother and sister to attend school, so when her father was released from his camp, the family decided to try to escape in hopes of a better life outside of Vietnam. When war broke out between North Vietnam and China, the North Vietnam government ordered all ethnic Chinese to leave the country. Though Ta's family was not Chinese, they pretended that they were and applied for papers to leave. "We could not speak any Chinese, so we just kept silent," she remembers. They abandoned their home, bribed a boatman with what remained of their money, and boarded a small boat with four hundred others. Their destination was anyplace that would take them in.

"The boat was very crowded," Ta remembers. "We did not have room to lie down on the boat, just sit. We had brought food and water for four days." Their boat was chased and fired upon by the North Vietnamese, but the refugees escaped harm. At the end of four days on the ocean, their boat approached an oil rig in the sea run by Malay-

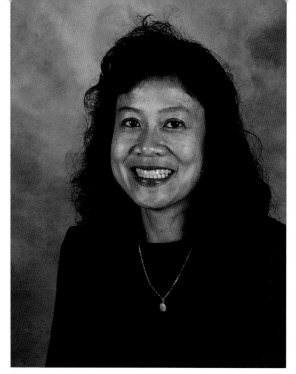

Psychiatrist Karen Ta escaped from Vietnam with her family by boat to a refugee camp in Malaysia before immigrating to the United States.

sian and American workers. The boat left the refugees with the workers, who gave them food and let them shower. "That night we slept out in the open and looked at the stars from the oil rig platform," Ta remembers.

After a year at an island refugee camp in Malaysia, with no electricity or running water, Ta's family immigrated to the United States. She was nineteen when she began her educational saga in Minnesota, attending college and medical school and then completing her cross-cultural fellowship in psychiatry.

In her present work as a psychiatrist for Westerners and immigrants alike, Ta feels special empathy for her refugee patients. "The Hmong, Cambodian, and Vietnamese all had to escape their countries," she says. "Each group is unique in what happened to them. The Cambodians had much more of a holocaust—people being massacred, losing family members, facing starvation. So they have a lot of [posttraumatic stress disorder] and experience more nightmares than do the Vietnamese. The Vietnamese are survivors of the camps."

Ta pauses for a moment, glances down at her hands, and adds, "Our staff has a special understanding."

Dr. Bruce Field

While he is not an immigrant refugee like his colleague Karen Ta, psychiatrist Bruce Field has impressive cross-cultural credentials: he worked for years with Hispanic patients at La Familia Clinic on St. Paul's West Side before joining the Center for International Health in 2002. Like Ta, Field sees patients every day who are profoundly af-

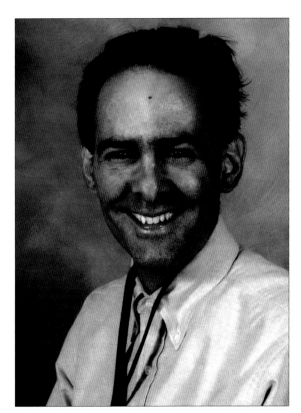

Psychiatrist Bruce Field previously worked with Hispanic patients on St. Paul's West Side.

fected by events in other parts of the world. Patients like Nadira, a middle-aged woman from Somalia who suffers from posttraumatic stress disorder.

Field remembers the day he and Nadira met in an examining room at the Center for International Health and she recalled for him the moment when her life changed. She was preparing dinner for her family when two crazed men wielding knives and rifles broke through the door of her home.

"Doctor, what happened next caused my soul to be broken," she told him.

The men ordered the family to stand in a circle. Nadira's father was standing on her left, her husband on her right. The men shot and killed her father, then they stabbed her husband to death with their knives. Her daughter was next. When Nadira tried to protect her, the men broke Nadira's leg.

"In my mind I still see my family standing around me, just like the moment before they were slaughtered," she told Field. "This picture never fades. It follows me wherever I go."

Nadira has become perpetually distraught and prone to sudden episodes of deep sorrow over her losses, which include not only her family but her language and her country. She has trouble sleeping, her body aches, and she has lost her appetite, not only for food, but for everything in life that gives pleasure. Field explains that, for people with posttraumatic stress syndrome, "the brain stays in a state of constant high alert, as if permanently under siege. There is never a sense of release or relaxation. A person's first concern, after experiencing overwhelming trauma, is that she may be attacked again. In order to protect herself she becomes obsessively vigilant, avoids all situations that remind her of her experience and constantly replays the tragedy in memory to understand it or, perhaps, to change the terrible outcome."

Field is hopeful about Nadira's prognosis and his ability to help her. There are treatments—a combination of medications and talk therapies—that can relieve her symptoms of depression and offer her encouragement. Field's role is to be a healing listener since telling the story is part of her treatment. But both he and Nadira understand that, despite her best efforts to explain to him the horror of what occurred, she will never be able to convey it all. And Field knows that, despite his efforts to imagine how it must feel to watch one's family be killed, and leaving the only country one has known for a completely different place, there will always remain, for him, an element of incomprehension. Yet as the relationship between psychiatrist and patient deepens, so does the potential for healing.

May Mua

Physician's assistant May Mua also sees the potential in nurturing relationships with her patients, many of whom also suffer from posttraumatic stress disorder and depression, particularly her Cambodian patients. But she sees drawbacks as well. "The trust I have developed with my patients is very important," Mua says. "Sometimes when you have developed a good relationship with a patient they won't go to see anyone else. I tell them that I have other coworkers who are good. Even though they have to wait a couple of weeks

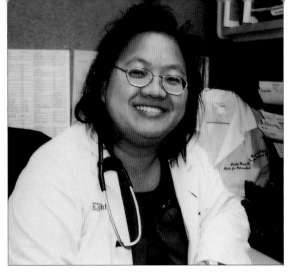

Certified physician's assistant May Mua was born in Laos.

to get in to see me, they prefer to wait. I am honored that they feel that way. But I don't want them to be too dependent on me, because it is not good for them."

May Mua understands the need for independence, but also the desire. "I broke tradition by going into a professional field," she says. "I was expected to be a good Hmong wife and stay home and take care of the kids. I wanted to have something to do for myself."

Mua was four years old in 1975 when her family emigrated from Laos to Seattle, Washington, and then to Fresno, California. Although her father never talked about his experiences in helping the United States during the Vietnam War, she knows that he was one of the Hmong farmers who rescued downed American pilots.

Mua grew up the oldest of five children in a traditional Hmong household. "I had a lot of responsibility," she remembers. "It is a Hmong expectation for the oldest. You take care of the family. It doesn't matter if you are a boy or a girl: if you are the oldest, you have more responsibilities." She looked after her siblings, and from the age of ten she accompanied her parents on their visits to doctors to translate for them. "Back then there weren't any interpreters to help, so the patients would have to bring someone in to translate," she recalls. "If you didn't bring someone in to interpret, the doctors would not see you."

Among the Hmong, a girl may marry as young as twelve and is considered an old maid if she is not married by the age of eighteen. Mua married at sixteen and became a mother a year later. She completed high school and earned her bachelor's degree in natural science from Fresno State College, all while juggling family responsibilities, including raising her own three children.

"Going to school and finding time to spend with my family was really hard," Mua says. "My in-laws were very supportive and they provided free daycare. Every day I dropped my kids off and they took care of them. I would come back late in the evening to pick them up. My husband worked full-time, and he would do the cooking and help with the household chores. That was not a Hmong custom either. My husband was just very supportive of what I was doing. "

Mua's career as a physician's assistant was determined after their two-year-old son, David, pulled a pan of hot oil onto himself and was badly burned. When Mua saw the excellent help little David received from the medical staff at the burn center, she decided that she wanted to become a person who could provide that kind of care. In 1996, after she and her husband, Tchamong, moved to the Twin Cities, Mua enrolled in the physician's assistant program at Augsburg College. After graduation, she earned her master's degree in physician's assistant studies from the University of Ne-

braska, then joined the staff of the Center for International Health in 2003.

About 30 percent of Mua's patients are Hmong. Like many of her Somali patients, she says, "the Hmong believe in going to the doctor only if they are sick. They don't understand prevention other than doing shaman ceremonies to help prevent illness in the family. . . . To come in for a physical when they think they are well and then be told they have high blood pressure or diabetes is overwhelming. If they are not in pain, they prefer not to come in." Her Hmong patients may think they are healthy, she says, but they "have a lot of diabetes, high blood pressure, and gout. It is related to their diet. The Hmong eat a high-protein diet, a lot of pork, beef, and chicken and rice at every meal. The younger generation is getting obese from eating chips and pop."

Because most of her Hmong patients are older and speak no English, Mua has an opportunity to educate them in their own language about their health choices. "Because I speak Hmong, they open up a bit more, tell me more about their condition and how they are feeling," she says. "Because I understand the culture, they confide things to me that they would not to another provider, like how they have tried traditional medicines and healing herbs or coining. Most of the herbs are OK, but some contain metals that are toxic. I have to be careful and check to make sure they are not taking any of the ones that could hurt them."

Her Vietnamese patients differ from other Southeast Asians in their health practices. "As a general rule, the [Vietnamese] stay on top of disease prevention," she says. "They come in for mammograms and Pap smears. They are not overweight, they eat more vegetables. Their main complaint is high cholesterol. They eat a lot of stir-fried food."

Somali women, who come to see Mua because they prefer a female provider, suffer from the same trio of complaints as her Hmong patients: diabetes, hypertension, and obesity. "Most of my Somali patients do not get any exercise," Mua explains. "It is not part of their lifestyle. The women are too busy taking care of six or seven children, cooking, and cleaning to have time to exercise." She refers them to the dietitian and urges them to get up an hour earlier in the morning to walk.

"A lot of my patients say that I am like their daughter, while others say I am like their mom. If they are not taking their medications and not doing things that are good for their health, I am a little hard on them. They understand that my goal is to help them to be healthy and get their problems under control."

This is succeeding with some of Mua's patients. "They come back to me and are so happy when they have lost five or ten pounds," she says. "They think I am the greatest, but I just provide the motivation."

Angela Kuria

Kenya-born nurse Angela Kuria understands all too well the importance of patient education at the Center for International Health, particularly when it comes to medicines. "Our patient clientele is non–English-speaking, so the medications, the therapies, are pretty foreign to them," Kuria explains. "We have elderly patients who have chronic illnesses and are on multiple medications,

and some of them are unfamiliar with what the medications they take are for. They know they have to take medications, but they are not sure which one is for which ailment. And they need to know that. It is very important.

"I take each medication, the pill, out of its package or bottle, stick it on a piece of paper, and write down, in English, the name of the pill so the patient will be able to identify it by color, size, and shape. Then I write down what the pill does and when the patient is supposed to take it. This information is translated into the patient's language. We have a sheet of paper that is written in different languages and divided into morning, noon, and night, on which we check off the date and times the patient is supposed to take the medicines. I translate the ones into French and Swahili for those patients."

Seated at a small desk in the clinic corridor, Kuria does phone triage on more than

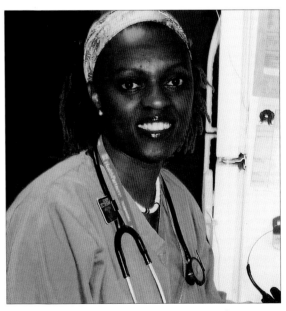

Angela Kuria of Kenya is the lead registered nurse at CIH.

eighty calls a day. "I prioritize the calls," she says in her British-accented English. "We get a lot of calls from clients at home who have various illnesses. They vary from coughs to chest pain. What we do is assess the patients—ask them questions to decide if they should come in to be seen right away or within the week."

Although the center has the option of offering home health care and home therapies, when a patient is sick, he usually wants to see a physician. "If the patient is adamant—'I have to see the doctor *now*'—we refer the call to the physician, who makes the final determination," Kuria says. "Our patients come from cultures where what the doctor says is law. Some of our patients believe the doctor can solve everything. If they need a letter for such and such, the doctor can do it. The doctor is held in high regard. It is not like the American culture where you can argue with your doctor, or not consider her the final say. Here, with our people, she is.

"Most of our clients, the Hmong and the Vietnamese and the Somalis, have gotten over their initial fear and have begun to trust their doctors. For patients coming from a culture where Western medicine is not used, everything Western is something to be suspicious of. Even in Kenya, anything Western is to be taken with a grain of salt or with suspicion. My grandparents would be that way, remembering colonialism."

Angela Kuria was born in Kenya to a single mother and attended British boarding schools in Nairobi. "Hospital Hill was a good school, a remnant of colonialism," she says. "Everything was British. English was considered the primary language. If you attended school in Nairobi, you learned English; but if you went to school in the coastal region of Kenya, Swahili was the primary language. Everything was taught in Swahili there. After the British left, we decided we should have a national language of our own. Since Swahili was spoken by quite a few of the different tribes, the government decided it would become the national language. It is taught in schools like you would teach French here."

After graduating from high school in Kenya, Kuria came to the United States in 1991 to enroll at the University of Wisconsin at Eau Claire. "My mother had a friend who went to the University of Wisconsin at Madison and she said great things about the school," Kuria says. "When I applied to various schools in the United States, UW–Eau Claire responded and offered me a scholarship." She had no idea just how different the cities of Eau Claire and Madison would be.

"Being in Eau Claire was a big culture shock for me," Kuria admits. "One of the things that struck me head-on was the number of white people. I had never seen so many white people in my entire life. I wasn't scared or anything; it was just different. It was difficult for the people of Eau Claire to relate to me as well. This was a little town. They had not been exposed to many people from Africa. I walked into a grocery store and kids just stared at me. One kid, I remember, asked her mother, 'Doesn't she shower or take a bath?' I didn't mind questions as long as I knew they were coming from a curious mind."

As part of their orientation, the freshmen students were invited to a steak night.

"Everyone was excited," Kuria remembers. "Steak night! It was held in this restaurant, and we were to sit with people we did not know. I was sitting at a table with two gentlemen and one other girl. One of the men asked me, 'So where are you from?'"

"I am from Kenya."

"Where is that?"

"Africa."

"It must feel strange," he observed.

"Yes. It feels strange being in a different country."

"No," he said. "It must feel strange to be wearing clothes."

"What do you mean?"

"Don't you wear leaves and things like that?"

Incredibly, the young man was not joking. "I was not upset with him," Kuria says. "It was pure ignorance. I encountered a lot of that. . . . I never felt at home, accepted, a part of anything. The African Americans who were at the University at Eau Claire would come for one semester only and then leave. We had maybe ten Africans, including African Americans, in a school of fifteen thousand. It was really hard."

Kuria made some close white friends, but felt fortunate to have another woman from Kenya as a roommate. "I do not know what I would have done if she had not been there," Kuria says. "If I feel uncomfortable, I tend to stay to myself. I don't go out and

break down barriers. She was different. She just let all of this stuff roll off her and continued to reach out. Where I became more quiet and angry and withdrawn, she was outgoing. Her outgoing nature helped me."

After Kuria graduated from college with a science degree, she moved to the Twin Cities and took a job as a secretary at the St. Paul Visitors Bureau. "I liked that, met all sorts of interesting people, went to a lot of events," she says. "It was a nice introduction to St. Paul." But her interests lay elsewhere. She wanted to work in the medical field and so went to nursing school.

"I absolutely loved it," she says. "It was more challenging than my undergraduate work had been. After I got my nursing degree and passed my boards, I started working [in Minneapolis] at Hennepin County Medical Center in the acute dialysis unit. They trained me really well, and I worked there for two years." Then Kuria began looking for a job that wouldn't require her to work every other weekend.

One of the places she applied was the Health Center for Women on University Avenue in St. Paul, where Pat Walker sees patients. When the nursing supervisor read her resume and saw that Kuria spoke English, Swahili, Kikuyu, and French, she told her, "You would be great at the Center for International Health." Kuria's application was forwarded to the center, but she did not wait for a call. She checked the center's Web site for openings and when one appeared a week later, she applied.

Kuria was hired in 2002. "I could not believe it," she says. "I am always saying, thank God that the clinic and I found each other."

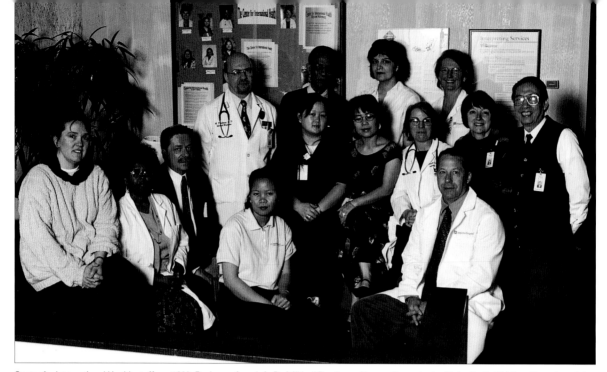

Center for International Health staff, ca. 1993. Back row, from left: Dr. Mikhail Perelman, Noeurn Ourng, Larisa Turin, Dr. Pat Walker. Front, from left: Sylvia McCalip, Dr. Fozia Abrar, Basil Ivanov, Christina Hang, Mai Mee Vang, Kim Fortney, Annette Frost, Robert Carlson, Kathy Lytle, Diem Nguyen.

Sharing the Wealth

Physician's assistant May Mua believes the Center for International Health "works" because "we all come from different cultures, so there is the understanding that everyone is different. We learn to help each other out. We pull together here because we all have the same goal: to provide good patient care. Though everyone does things somewhat differently, everyone understands that we are working toward one aim: trying our best to give good care to the patient."

To help codify and disseminate the principles of culturally competent care for patients with limited proficiency in English, Minneapolis-based Medtronic Foundation awarded Walker and the Center for International Health a three-year grant of $450,000 in 2003 to develop a twenty-hour curriculum for medical staff at Regions Hospital and throughout the Health Partners organization. The resulting program, called "Health in Any Language," is taken by physicians, nurses, pharmacists, and social workers.

Walker and Bill Stauffer, a former physician at the center, also designed a seven-and-a-half-week graduate medical education course in global health, which is offered at the University of Minnesota for resident physicians training in internal medicine and pediatrics. The course is the only one of its kind in the Midwest. In fact, it is one of only thirteen such programs in the world in this field, which include such famous programs as the London School of Tropical Medicine and Hygiene, the Liverpool School, Tulane University, and Johns Hopkins. The U of M course has attracted physicians from around the world, as well as nurse practitioners and physician assistants. Doctors completing the course are eligible to take the certifying examination from the American Society of Tropical Medicine and Hygiene and be certified in clinical tropical medicine and traveler's health.

The center's reputation for education and training was on a par with its stature in cross-cultural care. So in 2004, when the mayor of St.

Paul was told that a third of the Hmong refugees in the last remaining camp in Cambodia would be coming to Minnesota, he knew who to call for help. Pat Walker not only assisted Mayor Randy Kelly in assessing the refugees' resettlement needs, she started hiring more staff to deal with the anticipated influx. She hired medical assistants Shoua Yang and Mai Mee Vang, physician's assistant May Mua, and more Cambodian interpreters.

By 2005, those interpreters included Channy and Veera Som, the sisters who had first crossed paths with Walker twenty-five years earlier in the refugee camps during the madness that engulfed Cambodia in the 1980s.

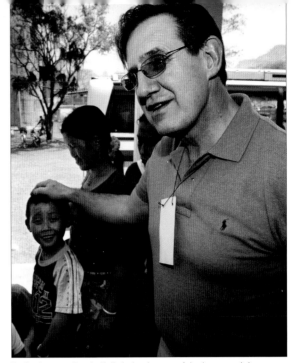

St. Paul mayor Randy Kelly helped some of the last remaining Hmong refugees in Thailand to resettle in Minnesota in 2004.

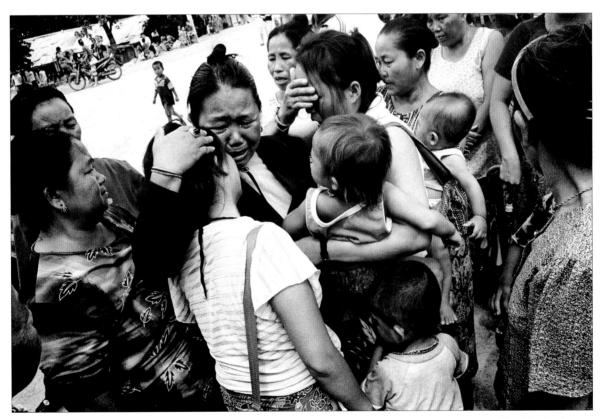

A mother leaving for America in 2004 hugs her sixteen-year-old daughter, possibly for the last time. The daughter was still waiting for clearance to leave the Wat Tham Krabok refugee camp in Saraburi, Thailand. Wat Tham Krabok was a 133-acre camp that held about fifteen thousand Hmong refugees from the secret war fought in Laos during the Vietnam War, when Hmong were recruited by the CIA to fight with the United States. The Thai goverment closed the camp in 2005.

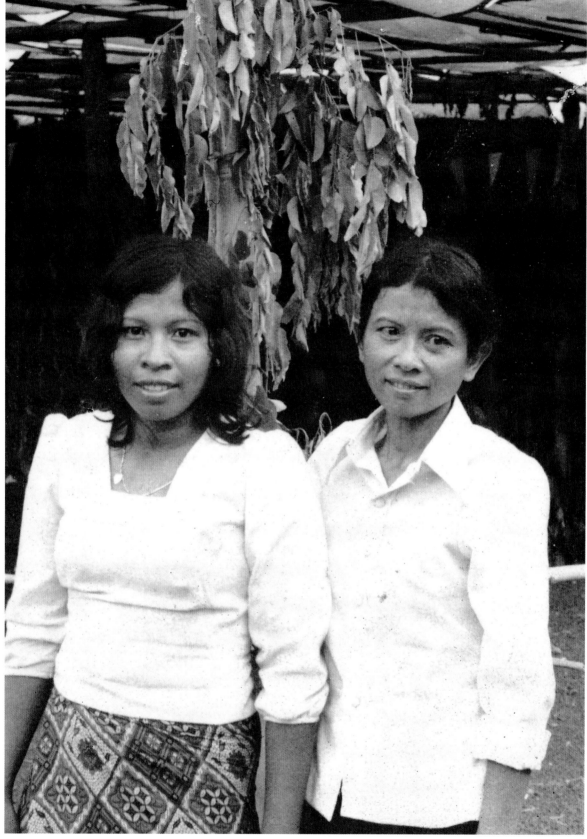

Sisters Channy (left) and Veera Som in the new blouses they bought for the Fourth of July celebration held by the American medical staff in the Ban Nong Samet refugee camp on the Thai-Cambodian border.

12: Veera and Channy

VEERA SOM WAS TWENTY-ONE years old and her sister, Channy, was fifteen in 1975, when the Communist Khmer Rouge overthrew the government of Cambodia. They were two of eight children, six girls and two boys, who lived with their widowed father in a small village in southwest Cambodia, about a two-day walk from the border of Thailand. "We lived in a small home, but we were happy," Channy remembers. "We had enough to eat—basically rice, fish, and, because we were poor, vegetables from the countryside. My father was a rice farmer and used a water buffalo or a cow in the rice patties and to move the rice. When I was young, I took care of the cow. There were no tractors or trucks back then, only the animals."

Their father, perhaps because he himself could not read or write, insisted that they and their siblings attend the primary and middle schools in the village. "I think we had a very civilized situation," Channy says. "All of my sisters and brothers attended schools and went on to the middle school. After middle school, students had to go to the city, about thirty kilometers away, for high school. My dad planned to send all of us to middle school and then high school in the city. He had to pay money to rent a place for us to stay."

It was a warm, sunny April 15 when armed Khmer Rouge soldiers appeared at the door of every house in Battambang, where Veera was completing her last year of high school. The soldiers ordered the people out, saying they had to "clean the city." Veera knew that something was terribly wrong. "People tried to take food and clothes, but the soldiers said, 'No, you can come back. Just go for three days.'" She grabbed some clothes and her textbooks. "I loved my philosophy book so much. My father had sacrificed to buy that book, and I carried it with me."

The soldiers forced the city's residents to walk in one direction only, but fortunately it was the way toward her family's village. "I walked all night and all day before arriving at my home," says Veera. "I was young and strong. Many people, older people and people carrying children on their shoulders, fell by the wayside." At home, she found her father returning from his rice field. With tears streaking his face, he told her how he had come upon dead bodies in the field and on the road. The next day, April 17, Khmer Rouge soldiers came to the village and began telling everyone they had to leave. Brandishing guns, they told Veera and Channy's family that they were to pack supplies for three days and to be out of their house within an hour. The girls bundled together clothes, blankets, and cooking utensils while their father filled a bag with rice and other provisions and tied it on the back of their cow. Under the hostile eyes of the soldiers, they abandoned their home.

When they reached the road, it was filled with throngs of people from their village and nearby towns, all herded by the armed soldiers in a single direction. Children, including Veera and Channy's two young brothers, were crying as the temperature hovered at 105 degrees. The soldiers threatened to kill anyone who stopped or stepped out of line onto the side of the road.

The villagers walked about ten kilometers until night fell and then camped under guard beside the road. The next day and the next the soldiers coerced them onward with blows and threats. After several days it became apparent that they were being forced to move into an area of Cambodia that was heavily forested. "My dad told us that the further we went into the forest, the harder it would be to find anything to eat, so he decided to just cut off," Channy says. When the soldiers were distracted, he guided his family along a trail that led to the outskirts of an abandoned village away from the main road. After a few nights of sleeping outdoors, he used tree branches and leaves to fashion a crude shelter for his family.

The Work Camps

At first the family lived on the rice their father had brought with them, but when it ran out, they began to starve, as did the other people around them. "People would not eat for three days," Channy says. "We were all starving. We ate anything we could find, but it never filled us up. People got thin, couldn't walk, got sick, and died every day."

As the Khmer Rouge became more organized, the soldiers took children from their families and placed them in work camps. "Siblings of the same age were separated . . . ," Channy remembers. "They took my older sisters away from the family to different teams and they took me away to another team. Even my two little brothers were taken away, but allowed to live near my father." Children as young as four were assigned to teams caring for cows or planting rice.

Channy's oldest sister, Kim, who had taken on the role of mother to her brothers and sisters, slipped away from her work team at night to make her way back to their father's camp. There he gave her the remaining family gold he had hidden and told her to buy food. Kim walked about fifteen miles at night to exchange the gold and some of the family's clothes for rice. "When we ran out of the gold and clothes, we began starving again," Channy says. The strain became too much for Kim. "She became ill and there was no medicine for her. She came home one night to my dad's shelter where, in 1976, she died of starvation. So my dad buried her in a place there."

In a desperate attempt to keep them alive, another sister took the two boys by night to another work camp, where an aunt and uncle were being held. If they were caught, they would be killed. "A relative hid the children, did not tell on them, and when they had some food they shared with them," Channy says.

Channy was confined to a work team a few kilometers from her father's camp. "In 1975 the Khmer Rouge were busy killing people and did not really have a structure set up yet, and there was a lot of chaos," she says. "They did not have me on all their lists, so I took advantage of that opportunity. . . . Every night I came to my dad or else walked to my sister's place. I became a fugitive. I was small and most of the time I could escape, hiding here and there. I was only about three feet, eight inches tall, and was very thin. I spent most of my time going to my sister's place, taking food to her and to my dad and going back to my team's location. I had to get back to my team before sunrise, so I did not get much sleep. By the time they woke up, I was back. "

Veera was placed on a team so far from her family that she did not see them for a year. But she learned from elderly people picking water grass that her sister Kim had died. Desperate to go home, she asked the woman who was the head of her team if she could have a day off to visit her father. Veera says she will remember the woman's answer for the rest of her life: "If you can make your sister come alive, I let you go. If you cannot and you come back, I will kill you."

The woman's reply so angered and depressed Veera that she resolved to kill herself. Having no knife or rope with which to commit suicide, she stopped eating. She refused to report for work, even when ordered, saying she was sick. She lay in a hammock slung between trees for three days before two people carried her in the hammock to the "hospital." "In the Khmer Rouge they did not have hospitals, just a place where they put the sick and gave them herbal medicine and some food," she remembers. "People were lined up side by side on the ground and many of them were dying. Nobody cared. When a woman close to my age died next to me, I decided to escape. Because they did not know who had died and who survived, they thought that I had died."

Veera knew the approximate location of her father's camp and began walking. When soldiers on bicycles appeared, she pretended to be picking grass and vegetables for her team. When she was too weak to walk any farther, she approached some elderly men who were drying herbs and asked them to let her stay with them. She explained that she had asthma and that her team leader had given her permission to find medicine to help herself. The old men let her stay. When she felt stronger, Veera continued her search.

When she finally found her family, the first to see her was one of her younger brothers. Having been told by others that Veera was dead, he stared at her and exclaimed, "Sister! Are you a ghost?" He ran to find their father. "They all thought I was a ghost and did not believe I was a live person," Veera says. "After they counted my fingers, they said, 'Yes, that is her. She has not died yet.'"

Veera stayed in hiding with her father for three days, then left to join a team where another sister worked. They pretended not to know each other, and Veera told the team chief that she had been sent there by her former leader. "You had to lie all the time. You had to be smart," she explains. "You had to pretend that you could not read or write. You could not have glasses, a watch, anything. Though I could read and write, I pretended I was blind. I never read to anybody. Our father had taught all of us to be honest, but in this situation we had to be clever. Our father told us to lie to survive."

Though her family had been moved about to various work camps over the years, all of them now knew where each of the others was being held. Recalls Channy, "We had to do whatever the Khmer Rouge told us to do. You had to do more than the best you could do to survive. We kept doing that and my dad told us to be really patient and one day this will change. I saw a lot of people killed. Their bodies were left in the field. They killed people by hitting them behind the neck and then cutting open their abdomens to get at their gallbladders. They believed that gallbladders could do something for them. Children and young people at meetings had to watch all of this. All the people had to watch. . . . I still have nightmares about it—the blood and how people died."

Escaping the Khmer Rouge

The change that Channy's father predicted came in 1979, when the Vietnamese invaded Cambodia. When rumors of the invasion spread, Channy, Veera, and their brothers and sisters slipped away one by one from their work camps to gather at their father's hut, where they made plans to escape. "My father said we had to have a quick plan. 'We can't go with the Khmer Rouge,' he said. We decided that when the Vietnamese came, we would flee."

For four years the family had no way to measure time, no calendar to keep track of the days. Yet Channy is certain that the Viet-namese arrived in the area of her father's camp on March 18, 1979. "The date was not important, but we still knew. One morning we just said, 'Let's go.' The Vietnamese were coming across the fields. The Khmer Rouge soldiers ordered us to come with them. We said, 'Yes, we will come,' but at the same time we planned to go another way. We had our plan. We walked and ran and walked and ran for hours. We kept going until six at night when we camped. A lot of people were there."

A neighbor family of Channy's father had prepared to flee with him, but they were caught and killed by the Khmer Rouge. An hour separated the fates of the two families.

Channy and her family began walking in the direction of their home village. It took them more than a month to get there. When they arrived, they found only a pile of wood where their house had once stood. "There was nothing there, but we were so happy," Channy remembers. "We just camped out and the next night we found a place to stay. It was April of 1975 when we left and when we came back home it was April also. It was very hot. Even though we had nothing, we had a completely new life." In four years the Khmer Rouge had killed an estimated 1.7 million Cambodians, one-fifth of the country's population.

The Vietnamese were occupying the family's home village and the Cambodians did not trust them. "My father still had five daughters and he told us to stay away from the Vietnamese," Channy says. "We did not speak their language, and even if we spoke a few words, we did not talk with them. We did not want to have anything to do with them.

"We were home about six months when the starving began again. People got sick in our village because there was not anything for them to eat. A few went for help to a camp on the Thai border, which was about two days away, but my dad said, 'Do not go.' My uncle and some other relatives went, but because we were girls, my father was afraid for us to go."

But as Veera's asthma worsened, she decided to make the attempt. Alone but for a guide, she walked for three days to reach the Ban Nong Samet refugee camp, where the American Refugee Committee was in charge of medical care. One ARC doctor gave Veera medication for her asthma, but because she missed her father and family, she returned to her Cambodian village. Within days she ran out of the medication and the asthma attacks returned. Veera realized that the only way she could survive would be to return to the border camp for treatment. She also knew that it was not safe for her to go back and forth. The border area was mined and infested with robbers who preyed on anyone moving through the area between the two countries. Despite the danger, Veera decided to return to the border camp, this time to stay. When Channy learned of her older sister's decision, she told her that, in a few weeks, she would follow her.

In deciding to leave their home village and family, Veera and Channy made a bold decision to take charge of their lives. Channy was now nineteen years old and could see that there was no future for her in her vil-

lage. Her school was gone, her friends had disappeared or been killed, her village was terrorized by foreign soldiers, and she faced the possibility of starvation if she stayed. Besides, she was intrigued by the stories Veera had brought back about the refugee camp hospital. Although it was run by the American Refugee Committee, it was staffed by Cambodian medics who had been trained by the foreign doctors and nurses.

The stories awakened Channy's old ambitions. "It had always been my dream to work in health care. That was my goal," she says. "I had no idea what an obstacle it would be to get there." If nothing else, she told herself, the camp would give her a glimpse of another world, a chance to experience life as it was lived outside the horrors she had known in Cambodia.

The morning she left home, Channy confided her plans only to her father. "If they know you are going, you can get raped or killed by the robbers," she says. "I walked with men who are guides. I avoided the mines by walking with people who had experience. We walked down the middle of the trail, a footpath about three feet wide. 'Don't step off the trail, never turn off,' they said." The trail crossed rice paddies and then entered a flat, forested area. People were coming and going on the path, some returning from the camp with food and smuggled items. Channy was in a group of about ten individuals. From time to time they encountered soldiers who stopped them at gunpoint and demanded bribes before letting them pass. "I was robbed many times," Channy says. "I told the robbers, 'I do not have anything. Take anything I have, take it.' These robbers were Vietnamese and Cambodian soldiers and we didn't know who else."

Ban Nong Samet

After two days and nights of walking on the worn trail, Channy arrived at the sprawling refugee camp of Ban Nong Samet. She found Veera, who had arrived only days before. Here, 120,000 people had created a makeshift village, lined up their rustic huts along newly created paths, and tried to recover from the trauma that had driven them from their homes.

When the two sisters registered with the camp administration, they received bamboo poles and a sheet of plastic with which to build a hut. They were given a ration card granting them each five pounds of brown rice a week, one tin of sardines and a sup-

ply of soy beans and vegetable oil every three months, plus twenty liters of water a day. Since they did not own a jar in which to store their water, they dug a hole in the ground of their hut, lined it with a piece of plastic, and poured their water in the hole. The nongovernmental organizations running the camp gave food only to women. The NGOs excluded men on the chance that they might be soldiers posing as hungry refugees to get something to eat. If the NGOs appeared to side with one army or the other, if they didn't maintain their neutral stance, they would be forced to leave the area.

From the day she arrived, Veera had been fascinated with the ARC hospital. Eager to learn English, she hung around to watch the staff to see how they did things. Soon she was volunteering in the dressing room. She

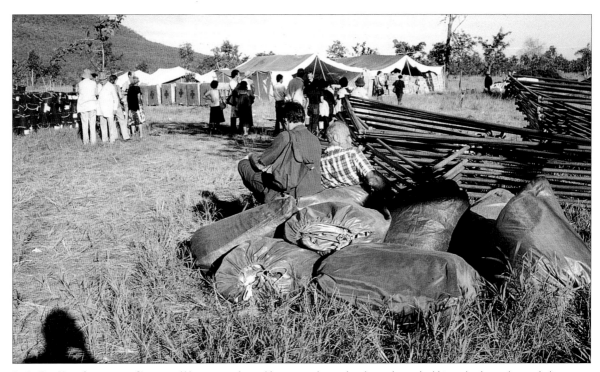

At the Ban Nong Samet camp Channy and Veera were given a blue tarp and some bamboo poles and told to make themselves a shelter.

cleaned people who were suffering from scabies, abscesses, and impetigo. She applied gentian violet to kill bacteria. She washed and hung up examination gloves that were used in the hospital and reused because they were in such short supply.

One day Mary Beth Brown, one of the ARC staff volunteers, asked Veera if she wanted to learn to be a medic. "I said yes. . . . Usually, before you can get in the medic class, you have to take public health nursing and another class. But she let me go directly to the medic class because I had volunteered in the clinic. She had taught me in the clinic how to give all the shots."

When Channy saw what Veera was doing, she told her sister, "I have to get in there too." Though the public health class already had sixty-three students, Channy talked the American teacher into letting her enroll. The lectures and lessons were presented in English using a Cambodian interpreter. "I learned English fast because I wanted to learn so badly," Channy says. She graduated at the top of her class.

One of the divisions of the camp medical service that needed assistance was obstetrics, but many of the newly trained Cambodian medics were fearful of working there because its director was reported to be very strict. "She was a very nice person, a wonderful person, but everyone was kind of scared of her," Channy said. "I wasn't, so I went to work in obstetrics and learned to be a midwife. The first week I only cleaned the instruments and observed—learned how to tie the cord, the basic stuff. Then I just began to do it. Later they sent me to a class, three times a week during the day. After that

I worked day and night delivering babies. We were busy twenty-four hours a day.

"After I had delivered 320 babies in the camp, my supervisor asked me to work only with the abnormal births and with patients who had issues with a normal delivery. I became a mentor to new midwives. I did not deliver the babies myself, but watched the new midwives to be sure they did everything properly, made certain the patient was safe, and that she understood what we were doing for her."

The Cambodian medical workers were volunteers, but as an incentive they were given an extra five pounds of rice a week. Veera and Channy felt fortunate to get double rations. For the first time in five years they had enough to eat.

The two became friends with the ARC medical staff. Veera and Channy met Pat Walker and Susan Walker when the sisters came through the camp on inspection tours. They also met Monica Overkamp, the nurse practitioner in the outpatient clinic and supervisor of the ARC-trained Cambodian medics who transported patients from the clinic to the camp hospital. The medics would come to Overkamp if they had a question about how to treat a patient.

"The Cambodians were wonderful people," Overkamp recalls. "Despite living in all this poverty, they wanted to learn as much as they could from us. Their big motivation was to learn English and have some contact with the outside world. They were so eager to learn. That is what was amazing: these people had so much adversity to overcome and they would come to class in their white

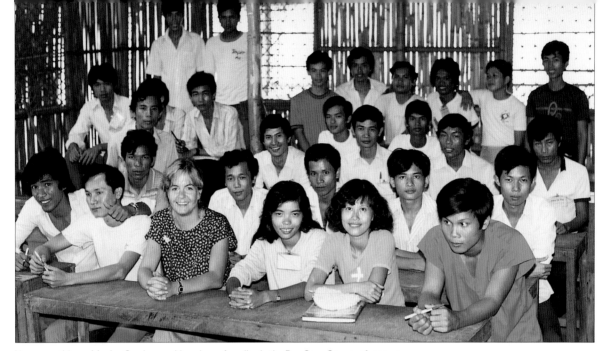

Nurse practitioner Monica Overkamp with a class of medics in the Ban Song Samet refugee camp.

shirts and blue jeans and their white tennis shoes. How can they be so clean? I wondered. They took a lot of pride in their work.

"Many of the students came from families that were educated, from Phnom Penh. But they had never had an opportunity to go to school themselves during the war. Anything they learned was self-taught. We showed them how to do spinal taps, sutures, put NG tubes down into people's stomachs, tie off blood vessels. They did a lot of minor surgery with a physician present. If there was no physician there, say, at night, they had to do it themselves—amputations, gunshot wounds, Caesarean sections. The midwives did them. They had to. The alternative was that the woman would die. These women, like Channy and Veera, were doing very complicated procedures they could never do in the States. They had high status in the camp."

Although Channy and Veera enjoyed their work and were no longer starving, they considered their life in the camp to be a little hell, only a small improvement from what it

had been like in the Khmer Rouge work camps. The outhouses at Ban Nong Samet were filthy and the camp swarmed with vermin and flies. There wasn't enough water. The camp was under constant attack from competing forces of the Khmer Rouge, the Khmer Serei, and the Vietnamese, which kept the refugees on the alert, ready to evacuate at any moment. During the years that Channy and Veera lived in Ban Nong Samet, the camp was moved many times to escape the fighting. When the foreign doctors left for the day, the camp was taken over by guards who robbed and raped the inhabitants.

Moving to Khao I Dang

In 1986, after seven years in Ban Nong Samet, Channy and Veera again decided to take control of their lives. As Channy explains it, "My life did not have anywhere to go. I felt as if I had no future if I stayed in the camp. I was happy to help other people, but I needed to take care of myself too. How could I ever get an education if I stayed in the camp? Moving to the Khao I Dang camp would be a step up for us. I never thought that I could come to the

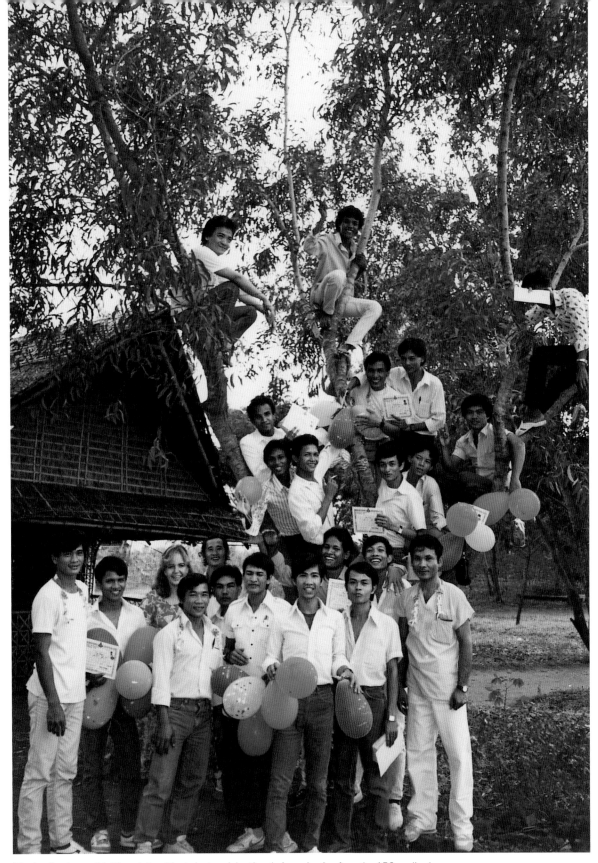

Monica Overkamp, third from left, with students celebrating their graduation from the ARC medic class.

United States, but I did think we should do something different, try something new."

The idea of leaving the security of the camp with its weekly ration of rice at first frightened Veera. Once outside the camp she and her sister would be illegal immigrants in Thailand and, if caught by the Thai police, put in jail. Thailand was no longer accepting refugees from Cambodia and the Khao I Dang camp itself was closed to any additional persons. For Veera, the risk of being robbed or raped on the way to Khao I Dang, and knowing that she and her sister could not legally enter the camp but would have to sneak in once they got there, was too frightening to contemplate.

Though Veera vacillated, Channy's mind was made up. She had had enough of the Ban Nong Samet camp and was willing to do anything to escape. She sold her remaining hidden piece of jewelry and with the money paid two guides to take them to Khao I Dang. One guide would lead Channy, who would walk the entire distance. The other guide would take Veera, who, because of her asthma, was promised that she would ride partway in a vehicle.

Channy was the first to leave, crawling on her stomach in the middle of the night under the barbed-wire fence that surrounded Ban Nong Samet, careful to evade the perimeter guards who would have shot her if she had been discovered. She was one of a group of eight escapees who, following their guide, walked for three days and three nights, hiding in the woods by day before crossing roads near Thai villages, taking quick naps, and living on the cooked rice they carried with them. One of their

party died on the journey and the body was left in the woods. About halfway to their destination they were attacked by robbers, who, in a pouring rain, made the refugees strip off their clothes so the robbers could check for hidden gold or money. The robbers stole the money Channy and the others had paid their guide, who then refused to take them any farther unless they promised to pay him again once they reached the camp. "I told him that I did not have the money now, but someday, somehow, I would find the money to pay him," Channy says. "I told him I knew a lot of Americans. And so he took us on."

The only way into the securely fenced and guarded Khao I Dang camp was through an enormous sewer pipe. Holding her breath and trying not to gag, Channy followed the guide through the fetid muck and water that rose to her waist. She pressed ahead through the dark pipe, which eventually passed under the camp boundary, to emerge inside the camp in a hut where, through a connection with the guide, they were hidden overnight.

Jeff Nelson, an ARC nurse at Ban Nong Samet, gave Veera additional money to bribe her guide to take her to Khao I Dang. Despite his help, she walked all night and rode only a short distance in an automobile. When she reached the camp, the guide bribed a Thai guard to make an opening in the wire perimeter so she could get in.

"We were illegally in the camp, and because the Thai government had ended its refugee program, if we were discovered we would be put in jail," Channy says. "Everyone had to have an ID badge and wear it all of the time. We did not have any badges, but there were some people who had left the camp to go to other countries and we were able to get their IDs. We had to learn a different name and memorize the number on the ID in case the Thai enforcement asked us any questions."

The sisters still faced the problem of where to live and how to get food. The problem was solved by Veera's asthma. Doctors Without Borders, a French NGO, put Veera in their hospital and Channy moved in with her, sharing her bed and food. "We went into hiding in the hospital," Channy says. "The doctors all suspected we were illegal, but we never spoke of it, because if the doctors knew for a fact we were illegal, they would be held accountable. They did not want to know and we did not want to tell them."

ARC nurses Monica Overkamp and Jeff Nelson and a Belgian doctor from Ban Nong Samet, all of whom traveled between the two camps, told their colleagues in Khao I Dang about the sisters' skills. Soon both were busy working for the doctors in Khao I Dang, and before long Channy had delivered another 330 babies. Nevertheless, they lived in constant fear that their presence would get the medical staff into trouble. Channy decided to quit for a while. "I ate by holding my bowl out when they gave food to the patients in the hospital," she says. "They gave food to the patients first and then some to me." She also hid in the leprosy ward "because the Thai guards never went into that building."

Veera, Channy, and their cousin Sarin were in the hospital one evening when Thai guards unexpectedly entered. Quickly the three hid themselves in the bamboo ceiling. "There were about twenty people up there," Veera remembers. "It was so dusty. I had my hand clamped over my mouth to keep from sneezing. When I climbed up I forgot my shoes on

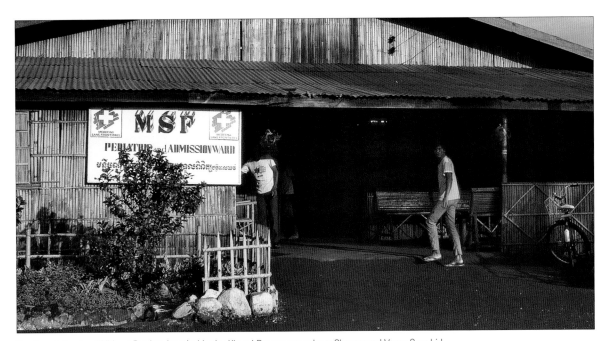

The French Doctors Without Borders hospital in the Khao I Dang camp where Channy and Veera Som hid.

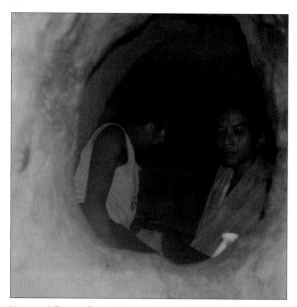

Veera and Channy Som at the entrance to the hole in which they hid at night to avoid the Thai camp guards.

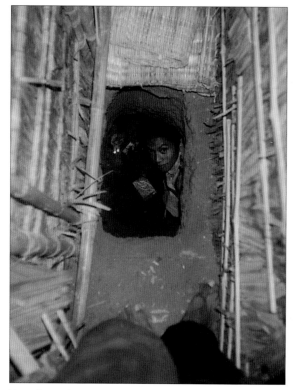

Veera Som, who had severe asthma, peers out of the tunneled entrance to the sisters' hiding place. The holes were hidden with beds, woven floor mats, or bundles of clothes placed over them. These can be seen at the sides of the photograph.

the floor. But the night staff saw them and hid them. The Thai guards were suspicious and kept moving their flashlights over the ceiling. After the guards left, the hospital staff told us it was safe to come down and find someplace to sleep."

After almost a year of clandestine living in the hospital, Veera decided "to get out of the hospital because I felt too ashamed." They had made friends with an elderly couple who agreed to help them by letting Veera and Channy tunnel a hole under their hut in which to hide. When Thai guards on patrol came around for inspection, the two women would drop in the hole until it was safe to come out.

"It was like a mouse hole," Channy says. "We would sit in there half the night. We would get in at eight at night and stay there until three in the morning. . . . They would put their bed over the hole and tell us when it was OK to come out. People risked their lives for us."

The foreign medical personnel knew what the women were doing. "The Thai solders went around looking for people who, when they heard them coming, would dive into these tunnels to hide," Monica Overkamp remembers. "Veera was using an inhaler and giving herself injections of epinephrine down in one of those crowded tunnels."

For twenty-one months Channy and Veera hid in the hospital wards and tunnels of the Khao I Dang camp and survived by begging food intended for patients. Then, in January 1990, their luck changed when Glenda Potter, an immigration attorney from St. Paul, came to visit her friend, Jean Jachman, an

ARC nurse in the Khao I Dang camp. When the ARC volunteers in the camp learned of Potter's profession, they told her that she had to meet Veera and Channy, who needed her help to get out, adding, "We will do anything we can do to help with the sponsorship."

Potter's friends had put her on the spot, but it was hard to argue with them. "People were afraid Veera was going to die because her asthma was so bad," she explains. "My friends asked me to help, so how could I say no?" Potter researched the sisters' options and learned that there was a little-used category in immigration regulations for people whose medical situations could not be taken care of in the camp. To apply under these regulations Potter had to show how Veera could get treatment in the United States and who would pay for it. "Veera's asthma was not expensive to treat," she says. "It was not like a person who needed heart surgery that was going to cost hundreds of thousands of dollars. What Veera needed was a different environment and some medicine."

The ARC staff at Khao I Dang rallied to support Potter's efforts. Jeff Nelson and Jean Jachman signed on as sponsors. Monica Overkamp and others in the camp wrote letters of support, as did Pat Walker, who had returned to Minnesota. There was still the problem of where Veera would live in the United States. Before she could get permission to immigrate, she had to have a guaranteed place of residence. This was a problem because all of Veera's American friends were working in the camp in Thailand. That left Glenda Potter. "I had just gotten my own house and was pretty happy

living alone and didn't know what it was going to be like," she says. Nevertheless, she signed the papers, stating that Veera could live with her.

The flurry of activity in the camp when Potter was interviewing Veera and gathering the detailed information she needed to file papers on her behalf did not go unnoticed by the Thai guards. The day Potter left the camp to return to the States, guards came in search of Veera. Fortunately, she had been warned and was safely hiding in her hole while the guards looked for her.

Veera had had another close escape. One day back in 1988, there was a staffing shortage on the night shift of the gynecology clinic and Pat Walker, knowing of Veera's training and experience, asked her to fill in. Because Veera was illegal, her name was not written on the clinic record. Suspecting that she was an illegal, a Thai coworker used the opportunity to steal supplies from the clinic and, to protect himself, reported Veera to the Thai authorities.

Walker learned of this in time to effect a rescue. "In a heavy rain, Dr. Walker came to find me at my hut and bring me to the hospital," Veera says. "There they put me in a bed with a fake IV. I will never forget. Thirteen ARC people helped me."

Shortly after that episode, Veera received word that she was accepted into the United States for medical reasons and, since she could not travel alone, that Channy had been given a visa so she could accompany her.

"My life changed two times," Channy says. "One was when I left home and the second was when Glenda Potter, the wonderful woman who changed my life, got Veera and me into the United States." Their family had no idea that they were leaving for America.

The sisters arrived in Minnesota in February 1990 to find the ground covered with snow and a crowd of people with TV cameras waiting for them at the airport. Both were exhausted, both had been airsick, and Veera's nose was bleeding. "When we came, we saw all the snow and all these people—it was overwhelming, a complete culture shock. What to do! What to say! They took us to a party at a home and there were Cambodian people there. They had a room for us, a bed—it was so amazing."

During the first week Potter had to keep the curtains in her house drawn because her two guests were suffering from jet lag and were disturbed by the brilliance of the sun reflecting off the snow. At first many things—loud noises, elevators—frightened the sisters. On their second day in the United States they began taking English classes.

Veera and Channy lived with Potter for three years. "It was really fun," Potter remembers. "My house was never so clean as when they were there. I had two cats at that time, and I knew Veera was allergic to them. I didn't know if my cats were going to have to live in the basement or not. But Veera increased her medicine a little bit and it worked out. Her asthma has gotten much, much better since she came."

When Channy and Veera moved out of Potter's house, they rented an apartment together and, while working to support themselves, also attended school. They went to Minneapolis Community College for two years to earn the prerequisite credits for entrance into college. For one year both took the nursing curriculum at Inver Hills Community College, but working full-time and relying on public transportation made it impossible for them to meet the demands of the program. Veera earned an associate of arts degree in liberal arts, while Channy transferred to Metropolitan State University and earned a bachelor's degree in human services. Channy also earned a certificate as a chemical dependency practitioner.

The End of the Exodus

In the years between 1975 and 1998 almost all of the refugees who flowed into the Thai camps from Laos had been processed to immigrate to other countries and had departed. By 2004 all of the official refugee camps in Thailand had been emptied and closed down. The rogue exception was Wat Tham Krabok, located an hour and a half north of Bangkok in central Thailand.

In fact, Wat Tham Krabok was not a refugee camp at all. All of its inhabitants were illegal aliens in Thailand. Many were elderly Hmong who had refused to leave the official refugee camps when others—like the Cambodians Veera and Channy, Monorom and Mony—had immigrated to the United States or to other countries. Over the next ten years about fifteen thousand Hmong filtered into Wat Tham Krabok, living there with no legal status and no medical care, barely surviving on the money their resettled relatives sent to them.

The Thai foreign minister gave the U.S. government an ultimatum: "Solve this problem for us. If you don't, we are going to get rid of these refugees." The United States agreed to take them in. A few weeks later Mayor Randy Kelly of St. Paul learned that five thousand new Hmong refugees would soon be coming to Minnesota.

Kelly immediately organized a team to go with him to Thailand to assess the condition of the Wat Tham Krabok refugees. Pat Walker accompanied Kelly, as did her brother-in-law, Jim Anderson, six Hmong Americans, and a few others. When she returned from the camp, Walker organized mass health screening at the Center for International Health for the Hmong refugees, bringing in physicians from all over the community to help. As she explains it, "We asked them to donate their time, but in exchange we taught them mental health and physical health screening for this population and connected them to the patients." Health Partners, the HMO that operates Regions Hospital, did not keep all the refugee patients, but referred many of them to the clinics where the volunteer physicians practiced.

Not unexpectedly, the increase in Hmong patients led to an increase in the need for interpreters—interpreters who would not only communicate the terminology of medicine, but speak the language of suffering. Interpreters like Channy and Veera Som.

In 2005, twenty-five years after Pat Walker first met the sisters in the Khao I Dang refugee camp, Channy signed on as an interpreter at the Center for International Health, while Veera became an interpreter at the Community University Health Care Center in Minneapolis. Neither of them could have foreseen a quarter of a century

earlier that they would again work in concert providing health care to refugees.

The days are gone when Dr. Neal Holtan, founder of the clinic that under Dr. Pat Walker became the Center for International Health, was stunned by the number of Americans he knew who had never met a Hmong, Somali, Russian, or Central American immigrant. Immigrants are now a sizable proportion of the U.S. population. Thanks to a diverse group of health-care workers in an obscure clinic in Minnesota, the precepts of cross-cultural medicine are now a recognized discipline. Medical personnel throughout the Western world apply the lessons learned in St. Paul, take the "Health in Any Language" course first financed by the Medtronic Corporation, and become certified in global health through studies now offered by medical schools throughout Europe and the United States.

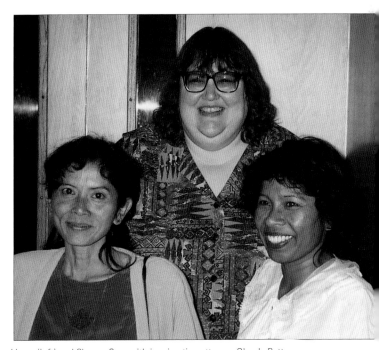

Veera (left) and Channy Som with immigration attorney Glenda Potter at Veera's 1994 swearing-in ceremony to become an American citizen. Channy became a citizen in 1995.

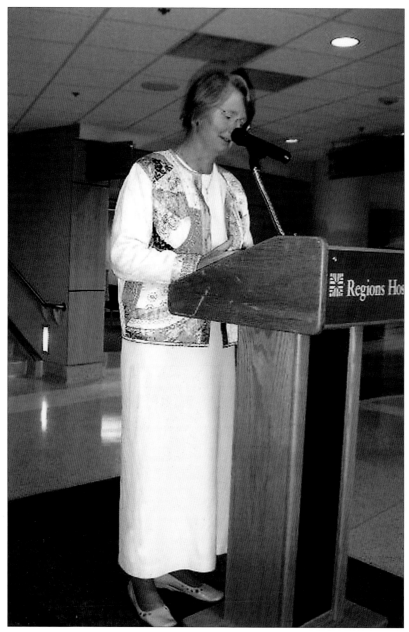

Dr. Pat Walker speaking at the observance of the twenty-fifth anniversary of the Center for International Health, Regions Hospital, 2005.

epilogue: health in any language

IT IS EARLY 2006, a few minutes before eight on a weekday morning at the Center for International Health, and already half a dozen patients are seated along a narrow corridor, waiting to be seen. In a few weeks the center will move out of Regions Hospital, its home of twenty-six years, and into a new outpatient facility it will share with another Health Partners Clinic.

In front of the waiting patients is a children's play area, decorated by the same framed Hmong tapestry that's been a fixture at the clinic for at least two decades. Many more languages—Khmer, Oromo, and Russian among them—have been added to the poster that once welcomed only Southeast Asian refugees to the center. A map of the world, covered with stickers marking the countries of origin of the center's patients, hangs next to a large frame holding photos of the center's nineteen staff members. In another hallway, thirty feet into the interior of the hospital and running parallel to the waiting area, is the operations center. The narrow space still doubles as an office, but the cafeteria table where Drs. Pat Walker, Neal Holtan, and Jim Jaranson once sat to write prescriptions and update charts has been replaced with several desks.

As the workday ramps up, the multicultural staff is self-directed. Lab technicians slide onto high stools to tap at computers and nurses answer blinking phones while physician's assistants and interpreters follow doctors into examining rooms. No one is giving orders. Each individual seems to know what to do, does it, and moves on. If there are hierarchical concerns, they are not apparent.

Today a new word, *jambo,* is being passed around the staff, who look and sound like a UN delegation. The Hmong and Cambodian interpreters try out their pronunciation of *jambo,* which means "hello" in Swahili, on Kenyan nurse Angela Kuria. Larisa Turin, the Russian nurse supervisor, smiles but keeps her eyes focused on her keyboard. Dialogues in Somali, French, and Spanish are interspersed with those in English, Hmong, and Cambodian. Snippets of Thai mingle with English as Dr. Pat Walker talks with her patients, while Russian dominates Dr. Mikhail Perelman's conversations.

When Perelman enters the corridor, he picks up a scrap of paper on the floor and moves a hydrangea plant from a work counter to a high shelf before he moves on down the hall. He stops in front of a door to

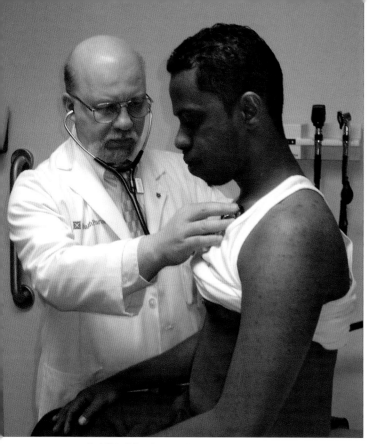

Dr. Mikhail Perelman with a patient.

which the day's schedule has been taped and silently fumes. Patients are scheduled to be seen every twenty minutes, beginning at eight o'clock. It's now 8:20 and Perelman's patient has failed to appear. If the patient shows up, Perelman will have to decide whether to squeeze him into the few minutes remaining of the scheduled time, spend the allotted twenty minutes and make other patients wait for the rest of the day, or send the latecomer home without seeing him. Perelman doesn't like any of his options. He understands the disparities immigrants face in getting health care, their lack of language skills and transportation difficulties. But this former immigrant has become a man of the West, for whom neatness, order, and time are essential ingredients of life. So he stands before the schedule, growling like the Russian bear he was when he began his medical career thirty years ago in the Soviet Union.

Pat Walker also scans the schedule. She too has been stood up by her first patient, but she takes it in stride. "Our patients are not driven by the clock, as we are," she calmly observes. Later in the day, when one of her patients arrives forty-five minutes late for his appointment, Walker debates whether to say something about the problems his lateness causes, then decides against it. "That's where the Asian in me comes out," she says. "Often the patient's only safe, enduring connection with the Western world is through people at the clinic."

Walker points out that, for non-English-speaking immigrants, the problems associated with access to health care are huge and frustrating. Many immigrants do not have cars and depend on family members or friends to bring them to their clinic appointments. Others who rely on public transportation might have to take several buses to get to the center. They may misunderstand or misinterpret times and directions. If they do show up at the clinic, they often cannot speak in their language with the doctor. The doctor may give them medicine, but they cannot read the label. If they have side effects, they stop taking the medicine until they can see the doctor again in three months for a twenty-minute visit.

It's not a new phenomenon. The underlying concept of culturally competent health care grew out of the American civil rights movement of the 1960s, when the United States became aware of the vast health disparities that existed between African American and Anglo populations. Reducing those health disparities is the major focus of Walker's work. National disparities data indicate, for example, that immigrant patients do poorly with diabetes, yet Walker is proud to have achieved the same outcomes with her immigrant patients who are diabetic as she has with her nonimmigrant, Western patients with diabetes.

"At the end of the day I ask myself, 'Did I help my patient live a longer life? Was his or her experience a good one today?'" she says. "We actually have measurements we can make that allow us to say, 'Yeah, we are doing that.' That is what makes me happiest."

People of color are a majority in forty-eight of the one hundred largest cities in the United States. In four states, minorities have become the majority of the population. By 2050, 90 percent of the nation's population growth will consist of Asians, African Americans, and Hispanics. Minnesota has always been home to immigrants—Germans and Scandinavians, Irish and Mexicans—but not until the 1970s and 1980s, when refugees began arriving from Southeast Asia, Russia, and Africa, did the practice of medicine in the North Star State clash so dramatically with the customs of non-Western cultures.

Thanks to the impact of the techniques and philosophy pioneered and developed at the Center for International Health, it is unlikely that today a court would order a spinal tap on a newborn as it once did for little Mai. Or would the issue of a patient's wish to have a tracheotomy tube removed go to the medical ethics committee of a hospital. More and more clinics and hospitals are hiring doctors and nurses who can communicate with patients in their own languages, providing interpreters and in-

structions about medications in many languages. Health care providers have become aware of the impact on health when cultural differences are not recognized and respected. As much as they are able, they strive to address each patient with compassion and cultural humility.

Cultural humility, Walker says, comes from a willingness to admit that Western medicine does not know all of the answers. Take the use of the herb artemether, she says. The herb had been used for two thousand years in China to treat malaria, yet only recently have its derivatives become the latest treatment for malaria throughout the world. Or consider the conversation that Dwight Conquergood, an anthropologist in Chicago, had with a Hmong shaman about the tools of his trade. On the shaman's altar were jaw bones of sacrificed animals, paper flowers, metal fragments, vials of herbal medicines—and a bottle of Western antibiotics. When Conquergood asked the shaman why the antibiotics bottle had been included, the traditional healer smiled and said, "Because sometimes it works."

An understanding that "sometimes it works" was in the minds of the nurses who stood aside while shamans kindled fires under patients' beds in the parking ramp of Regions Hospital. It motivated the aides who made sure that the drinking water of new mothers didn't contain ice. It enters Walker's mind when she goes into an examining room in her white coat, sits knee to knee with one of her Hmong patients, disregards the bruiselike marks of coining on his arms, and leans forward to ask, "What is your problem? How can I help you?"

Practicing Culturally Competent Care

Wearing bright blue scrubs, Christina Hang perches on a high stool by the waiting-room door and checks the computer for the name of Walker's next patient. Hang is Walker's Cambodian medical assistant, whom Walker calls *ohn,* meaning "younger sister" in Khmer. When the patient arrives, Hang ushers her into one of the white-walled examining rooms. Many if not most of the immigrant refugees that Walker sees at the center have multiple health problems. While some complaints may seem routine, the source of their pain is not.

Seventy-year-old Mrs. Gomez, a first-generation Mexican American who has diabetes, is making her first visit to the center. Dressed in a white skirt and floral print blouse, she speaks English with a pronounced Mexican accent. Walker tells her that her blood sugar numbers are low enough that, if she controls her diet and exercise, she won't need pills or insulin for many years. She also gives Mrs. Gomez the good news that she does not have hepatitis B, an ailment common among people of Mexican descent. However, her cholesterol is high, so Walker wants her to increase her Lipitor dose to 20 milligrams.

The two women sit in a companionable silence for a few moments before Mrs. Gomez decides to confide her other difficulties to Walker, including financial burdens incurred after her hysterectomy some years ago. Her severe allergic reaction to the latex gloves used during the surgery caused her medical bill to soar. Insurance covered only 80 percent of the expenses, so she's been paying off the remaining debt ever since. She has only a few more payments to go, she tells Walker with pride.

Then Mrs. Gomez adds that she has asthma and uses her great-grandson's nebulizer from time to time. Walker asks to see the inhaler she's been using, notes that it does not have the proper extension tube Mrs. Gomez needs, and tells her, "We'll get it for you." Mrs. Gomez then admits she has eye problems. Another clinic prescribed eye drops, but they cost more money than she could afford. Walker promises to get someone at the center to help Mrs. Gomez fill out the necessary paperwork to get the eye drops at a reduced rate.

Thirty minutes after the two women say goodbye, a distraught Mrs. Gomez is back, trying to get someone's attention outside the examining rooms. Mrs. Gomez explains to an aide that when she picked up her prescriptions at the pharmacy, the bill came to $400. She thought she was on a health-care program that covered her medications for $35. The aide calls social worker Kathy Lytle, who promises to track down the other social worker Mrs. Gomez previously worked with and have her call the patient. Lytle suspects that her colleague will probably refer Mrs. Gomez, who has no insurance, to RX Connect, a state and federal program for which she may be eligible. Whether Mrs. Gomez can navigate the paperwork involved in meeting the program's requirements, however, is questionable. She goes home without her medication.

Walker next sees Mrs. X, a sixty-year-old Cambodian woman who also has diabetes. In the room with her are her daughter, who works for an insurance agency, and Cambodian interpreter Paula Keo. Walker pulls up a stool and opens the conversation. She keeps her eyes on her patient while the interpreter translates. As soon as the interpreter stops talking, Walker picks up the conversation. After a few minutes, the process of speaking and interpreting becomes seamless.

Mrs. X tells Walker that she and her husband fled the Pol Pot regime in Cambodia in 1979 and lived for four years in a refugee camp on the Thai border, where her daughter and two other children were born. The family then moved to a camp in the Philippines for five months before immigrating to the United States. Walker and Mrs. X compare dates and discover that they were in the Khao I Dang refugee camp at the same time. Walker asks Mrs. X if she still has nightmares about her experience with the Khmer Rouge. She answers yes.

Walker tells Mrs. X that, despite her diabetes, she will be able to live a long life if she takes the medicine that Walker prescribes. Mrs. X does not understand why she has diabetes since she does not eat sweets. Walker takes time to explain that the rice Mrs. X eats is a carbohydrate that converts to sugar in her body. She also makes a note to send Mrs. X to a dietitian to help her with meal planning. Walker then asks Mrs. X's daughter how her mother gets to her clinic appointments. The daughter says she uses sick leave from her job to bring her mother in. Out in the hall, Walker asks her assistant to work with Kathy Lytle to arrange transportation for Mrs. X in the future so her daughter will not jeopardize her job by taking off too much time.

Waiting for Walker in the next examining room is Mark, a thin young refugee from Liberia whose family is descended from American slaves who returned to Liberia after the U.S. Civil War. Mark has sickle-cell anemia, a hereditary blood disorder. When an African inherits the gene for sickle-cell anemia from one parent, it protects him from contracting malaria. If the defective gene comes from both parents, however, it causes sickle-cell anemia, which results in severe joint pain and, too often, an early death.

In barely inflected English, Mark tells Walker that he was living in Monrovia with his siblings in 1992 when rebels began a systematic slaughter of the capital city's inhabitants. He and his four brothers and sisters decided to flee to the United States, where their mother was already living. Tragedy struck the night before they were to depart, when Mark's gravely ill niece and nephew died. Early the next morning, the family had no choice but to hastily bury the children in the yard, abandon their home and possessions, and make their desperate escape from the city. They walked for three weeks, and were twice threatened and almost shot by gun-wielding bandits, before reaching safety. Though it took a year, their mother successfully completed the paperwork for the family to immigrate to the United States.

Mark relates his story dispassionately, as if recounting a dream that doesn't yet make sense. He then tells Walker that he is studying computer programming and Web page design at the University of Minnesota. To pay his tuition, he works in a restaurant from eight in the morning until midnight. Walker knows that immigrants often arrive in the United States healthy, but can become ill from psychological stress, poor eating habits, and a lack of exercise. She praises

Mark for managing his sickle-cell anemia so well, despite his grueling schedule.

Next on the schedule is Judith, a vivacious young Haitian who has been in the United States for about ten years. She too has sickle-cell anemia. She was recently hospitalized for eight days with pneumonia, a condition that can accompany the disease, and is having severe pain in her joints as well as occasional paralysis.

Judith's story is a violent one. She was a supporter of Haitian president Jean Bertrand Aristide, a Catholic priest, when he was overthrown in September 1991. Judith and her brother worked with a group in her church that supported the return of Aristide, who was reinstated as president under U.S. protection in October 1994. But when their political activity was discovered, Judith and her brother were sent to prison, where Judith was raped. Her parents secured her release only by paying the police a large bribe.

Judith went into hiding at the home of friends, but knowing she was risking their lives as well as her own if she stayed in Haiti, she applied for political asylum at the U.S. Embassy. When it was granted, she boarded a plane bound for the United States, but was not told where it would land. She found herself in Minnesota, where she was met by a cousin, who housed her for one week and then told her she had to find a place of her own.

Judith is struggling to get by. She was recently laid off from a job she had held for more than nine years. She shares an apartment with two others; she pays $150 in rent from the $250 she receives in welfare

each month. A friend is making her car payments for her. Judith's psychological stress is compounded by the fact that, since leaving Haiti, her parents and several siblings back home have died, some from sickle-cell anemia. Judith hopes to attend school to become a medical records technician, a job that will place less stress on her body. Walker suggests that she do deep breathing exercises every day and asks her to come back in one month for a chest x-ray.

A Russian immigrant named Sima greets Walker with a loud "Welcome!" when she enters the examining room. Sima has learned to speak English quite well since she and her husband immigrated to the United States from Kiev in the wake of the Chernobyl nuclear reactor accident in April 1986. Walker looks for signs of lymphoma among her patients from Russia. Four have developed the cancer after being exposed to radioactive fallout from the Chernobyl incident. So far, Sima seems well.

That's not the case for Walker's next patient, a young refugee from Ethiopia named Marwan whom Walker suspects has tuberculosis. Fifty percent of all immigrants carry the TB bacteria, if not in their lungs, then in their bones or other organs. Though Marwan's earlier test for TB came back negative, a scan of his lungs shows the presence of the infection.

Marwan arrived in the United States in 1989 as a deckhand. Wearing tattered clothes as a disguise, he jumped ship while it was docked in a Delaware harbor. He waved down an African American taxi driver and explained that, despite his ragged appearance, he had money not only to pay for the cab ride but to buy decent clothes. Their first stop was a clothing store, then the airport, where Marwan bought a ticket to Minneapolis, where his sister lived. He has since obtained a visitor's visa and applied for political asylum.

In broken English, Marwan tells Walker about his symptoms. Although he doesn't have a classic TB cough, he sweats all of the time, which is another common sign of the disease. Walker wants to schedule him for a bronchoscopy, a procedure that involves putting a scope down the throat and into the lungs. Marwan balks at her description of the uncomfortable procedure and resists proceeding with the test, but he finally agrees to it after Walker assures him he will be sedated. She asks her assistant to walk with Marwan down to the pulmonary clinic to make his bronchoscopy appointment.

In the next examining room, a heavy-set woman from Pakistan named Mrs. Bafat greets Walker with a happy smile and begins talking at once. Mrs. Bafat (and, before his death, Mr. Bafat) has a long history with the center and considers Walker to be her friend. The Bafats and their six children left their affluent life in India in 1986 to come to Minnesota. Mrs. Bafat has a bachelor's degree in history and English from a Pakistani university and her husband was an attorney. All of their children have earned college degrees in the United States and are pursuing professional careers.

Mrs. Bafat suffers from diabetes, but has been careless about controlling her blood sugar. She claims that her blood monitor doesn't always work, but she has also ignored Walker's advice to get more exercise.

As if to head off the questions about diet and exercise she knows Walker will ask, Mrs. Bafat addresses her major concern: "Will I get a heart attack and die like my brother?" Her brother and father have died in their sixties from heart disease, she says, and she's worried she may be next. She adds that her blood sugar numbers are elevated because she is still grieving for her brother. She then shows Walker an insect bite on her right arm, fearful it may be a sign of impending heart trouble.

Walker gets to the point: how is Mrs. Bafat managing her grief? The patient explains that her family does not want her to talk about her dead brother because they believe this will make her ill. "Talking about him cannot bring him back, so they don't allow me to talk about him," she complains. Walker agrees that there is a connection between grief and health, and considers sending Mrs. Bafat to the center's psychologist for counseling. Instead, she explains that the best thing Mrs. Bafat can do for her heart is to keep her blood sugar under control and lose weight by walking. She tells Mrs. Bafat that doctors are now recommending sixty to ninety minutes of walking six days a week. Mrs. Bafat looks doubtful and replies that she becomes breathless when she walks quite slowly for twenty minutes. Walker orders a stress test for Mrs. Bafat and refers her to a diabetes counselor for help with her diet.

Walker's last patient is the most challenging. Hassan, a Somali in his late forties, has been referred to the Center for International Health by his infectious-disease specialists with the notation that he is "failing to thrive." The specialists believe that Hassan has tuberculosis, but he won't allow them to do a bone-marrow biopsy to confirm their suspicion. (Many times the TB bacillus can be grown from bone marrow when it cannot be found in other places in the body.) Meanwhile, Hassan has lost thirty-five pounds. He is anemic, runs low-grade fevers, and has pain in his hip. Something is preventing him from accepting his doctors' advice. Frustrated, they have referred him to the center.

As Walker talks with Hassan, she learns that he not only has studied engineering, but that he spent eight years in the Soviet Union. She then asks internists Mohamud Afgarshe and Mikhail Perelman to join her in her meeting with the patient. After her colleagues exchange pleasantries with Hassan in Somali and Russian, they say, "We think you have tuberculosis. You must get a bone marrow biopsy. It's really important that you do this because if you don't, you will continue to get worse and you will lose more and more weight."

Hassan agreed to the biopsy. It confirmed the presence of tuberculosis, which the doctors were able to treat. Walker believes that her team was more successful with Hassan than his infectious-disease specialists because of the center's cross-cultural approach with him. "We were impressed with Hassan and the fact that he spoke Russian, and we treated him very respectfully. He, in turn, trusted us. The infectious-disease doctors had figured out the diagnosis, but they weren't getting anywhere with Hassan because of the cross-cultural issues."

Biological Bridges

The concept of "immigrant medicine" is obsolete, a holdover from the days of Ellis Island, when foreigners arrived in a new country expecting to stay in one place the rest of their lives, says Canadian physician Brian Gushulak, who, like Dr. Louis Loutan of Geneva, organizes international conferences on global health care access. Twenty-first-century immigrants spend months or years in countries that serve as way stations, often moving to a third or even a fourth country, Gushulak says. Some, after decades of dislocation, return home. Under "rights of movement," residents of what were once European colonies in Africa and the Caribbean now move back and forth between the nations that had once colonized them. Vast pools of labor flow continuously across the globe.

The United Nations estimates that 191 million people now live in countries other than those where they were born. If all of these people lived in one place, they would constitute the sixth or seventh largest country in the world. "Migrants have long been a reality in every country," Walker observes, "and we need to learn better ways to deal with population movements around the world."

People moving around the globe are biological bridges, bringing with them ailments once considered specific to particular regions. Diseases such as malaria are no longer isolated to the tropics. As Walker discovered with the *Strongyloides* worm, U.S. health-care providers have to be aware of the peculiarities of intestinal parasites once found only in isolated areas of Asia.

Sensitivity to issues of culture and the special problems of immigrants is no longer exclusive to clinics like the Center for International Health in St. Paul, which

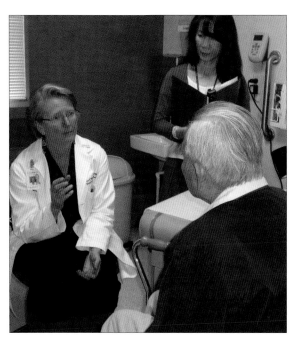

Vietnamese interpreter Malinda Christopher translates Dr. Walker's comments while Walker maintains eye contact with her patient.

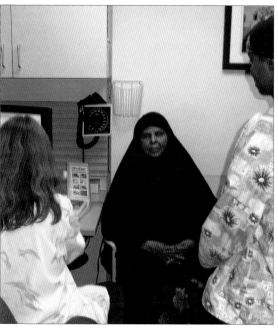

Ayan Ali, on the right, interprets for a Somali patient and nurse Ginny Nierad. Ali, who is a certified medical assistant, does not usually interpret but was filling in.

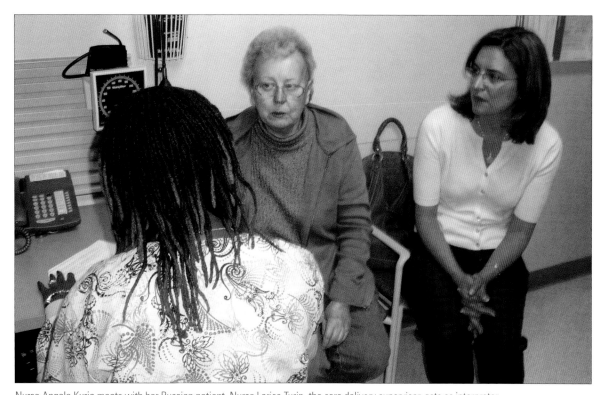

Nurse Angela Kuria meets with her Russian patient. Nurse Larisa Turin, the care delivery supervisor, acts as interpreter.

accommodates approximately twenty thousand patient visits a year. But the center continues to be one of the concept's chief advocates, thanks to Pat Walker, now one of the most internationally recognized experts on immigrant health in the United States. Walker addressed an international conference in August 2006 in Geneva, Switzerland, where eleven hundred participants from all over the world discussed global access to health care and how to create immigrant-friendly hospitals in both Europe and the United States.

Such facilities already exist. At Oakwood Hospital in Dearborn, Michigan, a city with a large Arab population, nurses point the beds of Muslim patients toward Mecca. Clinics associated with Maimonides Medical Center in New York, long known as a Jewish hospital, have painted their white walls shades of yellow and pink because their Chinese patients associate white with death. Lutheran Medical Center in Brooklyn, New York, has a mosque on site and runs clinics aimed at Caribbean and Korean immigrants.

Making such accommodations does not always go smoothly. "In each culture that we're dealing with, there are different ideas, family values, and beliefs, whether about medicine or life in general," says Virginia Tong, a vice president at Lutheran Medical Center. She acknowledges that cultural differences make delivering comprehensive health care more challenging. Like the Hmong, the Chinese believe that drawing blood for tests drains a person's life force and so are reluctant to allow it. Physicians who see immigrants from India must be aware that those patients have disproportionately high rates of hyperten-

sion. Physicians seeing babies from Bangladesh must be alert for signs of measles in the infants.

Medical professionals now agree that the single most important factor in serving patients with limited English proficiency is the presence of an interpreter. Barriers of culture and language fall when there is a Diem or a Monorom, a Channy or a Veera who becomes a partner with a physician to bridge the gap in understanding medical treatment. On September 15, 2006, the New York State Health Department announced that it will require state hospitals to provide skilled translators for patients with a limited understanding of English. The new regulations clarify who can act as a translator, require hospitals to appoint a language coordinator, and mandate that each patient's primary language be identified in medical records.

Walker and other Western-trained physicians who practice culturally competent health care include in their own diagnostic and treatment repertoire those procedures or substances not generally used in Western treatments. These doctors recognize the power of cultural beliefs, respect their patients' need to honor centuries of traditions, and remain flexible in bending the conventional model of Western medicine to work more successfully with their patients in treating their ills.

"Here, the doctors will encourage practices such as 'coining' if they are something the patient believes in and will do no harm," says Angela Kuria, the lead nurse at the Center for International Health. "Allowing this in conjunction with Western medicine validates the patients and makes them and their culture feel important. When you come here from a different culture, you soon notice that many parts of your own culture have begun to diminish or go away. These are personal customs that our patients hold on to and feel that they must not be taken away from them.

"Because most of us in the center are immigrants, we feel this sense of connection. We understand each other. Regardless of where we come from, Thailand or Russia or Africa—totally different worlds—we can relate to each other because we are immigrants. We understand that we have differences. We don't feel that we have to be like each other. This is so wonderful, like a deep understanding. I really treasure that. You feel at home."

Kuria says that the Center for International Health staff feel this same sense of connection with their patients. "It helps that we have doctors from our patients' own communities," she says. "I think that is the best thing that has ever happened in medicine, especially for immigrants. Nothing is lost in translation or in interpretation. Little things, nuances, where a patient can say something that, if it is translated literally, can mean something totally different, are not lost. Our patients are treated with understanding by people who are acquainted with where they came from, who understand their culture. If a patient comes in and says she has tried everything to get well, including going to a spiritual doctor for 'coining'—something the Hmong do—the physician will understand what the patient is talking about. The doctor will never say, 'Why did you try that? Don't you know it won't help your diabetes?'

"When a health care provider has had similar traumatic experiences as his patients, the

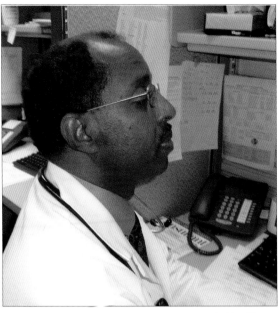

Dr. Mohamud Afgarshe transcribes patient notes in his office.

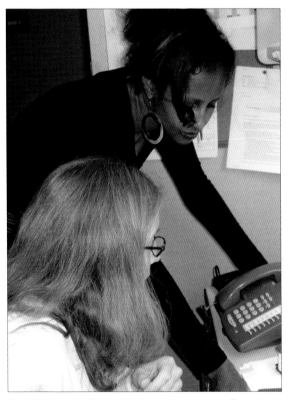

Somali interpreter Fartun Wardere interprets nurse Ginny Nierad's instructions on medications to a patient in a phone conversation.

benefits can be huge. When a patient says, 'I am not able to sleep at night because I went through all of this' and the provider has experienced something like it, or knows others who have, he can relate. He can see the dramatic effect that experience is having on the patient, even though the patient is now safe in this country. The provider understands that patients do not automatically shut off their anxiety, do not automatically feel safe when they come here."

For Walker and her fellow physicians, their personal experience in divergent cultural settings has provided training as valuable as their formal medical rotations. "You can talk about compassion," she says, "but the way you really learn it is to sit next to someone as he spends the entire night telling you the dreadful things that happened to him."

Adds Kuria, "Here at the center we have our own little world in this big strange world we are in, which we are all trying to understand. It is a totally different working environment. I have worked in hospitals with Americans, and there you are constantly explaining yourself or trying to fit into that world. You get a lot of 'I'm sorry, I don't understand what you are saying.' Here, it does not matter how you speak because everybody is going to try very hard to understand you. That is priceless."

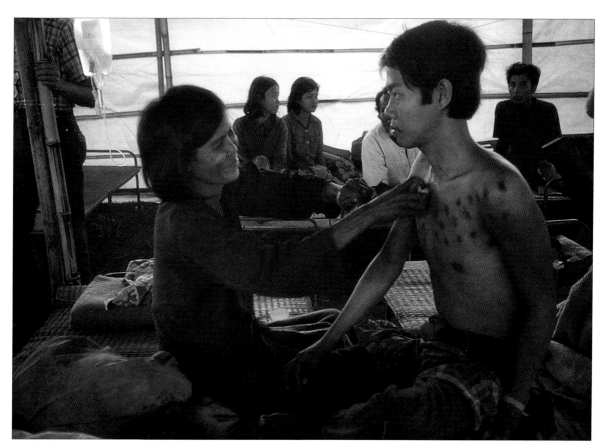

This youth is being treated in Thailand with a folk remedy of pinching the skin. The procedure is similar to "coining," the act of rubbing coins on the skin to draw out a fever.

"my heart it is delicious"

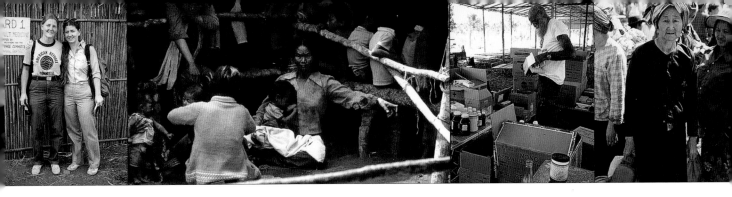

appendix: where are they now?

Center for International Health

On May 1, 2006, the Center for International Health moved into its new home at 451 North Dunlap Street in St. Paul, in an outpatient facility it shares with the Midway Clinic. The center was the last of the primary-care clinics to move out of Regions Hospital, whose focus is now surgery, trauma care, and inpatient rather than outpatient care.

American Refugee Committee

Back in 1979, in its first full year of operation, the American Refugee Committee did not have the money to bring its medical volunteers back from the Thai refugee camps. The organization now operates with a $28 million annual budget and conducts a dozen programs around the world, from Darfur and the Sudan to Guinea and Kosovo. It may be thought of as small when compared to the major nongovernmental organizations housed in New York and Geneva, but Minneapolis-based ARC has racked up an impressive and enviable record.

In 2005, after Bill Clinton and George H. W. Bush visited ARC's Fishing Boat Restoration Project in Thailand—the only relief project the former U.S. presidents visited in that country—they awarded ARC $1 million. It was the first relief project to receive funding through the Bush-Clinton Houston Tsunami Fund. ARC also received a $1 million grant to provide health care to survivors of the 2006 Pakistan earthquake, thanks to an initiative led by the elder President Bush.

Reader's Digest, Money, and *Worth* magazines all have classified ARC among the nation's best charities. ARC also has earned *Charity Navigator*'s highest ranking of four stars for its financial health and organizational efficiency. "ARC is small in size, but very effective," adds Karen Johnson Elshazly, former director of operations. "We are admired. The values inherent in the Midwest have made us special."

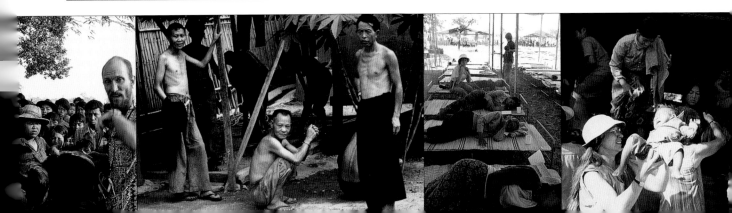

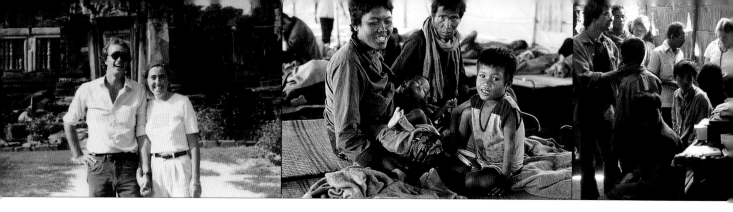

Dr. Fozia Abrar

Abrar is director of Health Partners' Occupational Medicine Clinic.

Elizabeth Walker Anderson

After working for several years as the cross-cultural supervisor at the Center for International Health at Regions Hospital, Anderson decided to become an attorney. While a student at the William Mitchell College of Law in St. Paul, she received the top award for community service for her work on immigrant legal issues. She is community relations director at the Minneapolis offices of Thrivent Financial for Lutherans, the nation's largest fraternal benefit society. She and her husband, Jim Anderson, who is the human services planner for Ramsey County, have two sons.

Neal Ball

Ball retired from the American Hospital Supply Corporation in 1985 and continued as chair of the American Refugee Committee through its years of explosive growth until 1991, when he became ARC's honorary board chair. Still living in Chicago, Ball remains active in international affairs. He is a member of the National Committee for UNICEF and serves on the boards of a medical ethics foundation in Barcelona, Spain, and a New York foundation that provides medical-school scholarship aid to minority students. He stays in touch with Phunguene Sananikone, who lives with his reunited family in New York City, where they own and operate a limousine service.

Yong Yuth Banrith

After Banrith left the Khao I Dang refugee camp in Cambodia, he went to Switzerland, where his eldest brother was serving as a diplomat, and attended a gourmet chef school. Upon graduation he responded to the urging of Pat Walker and Barbara Huwe to come to Minnesota, where he opened a French restaurant called Suzette's, named after Walker's sister Susan. In 2003 Suzette's, which is located southwest of Minneapolis in the town of Jordan, was named the "best French restaurant in the Twin Cities" by a local magazine.

Banrith and Walker are related by marriage. Walker's cousin David, the son of her mother's sister, married Saynearirath, a cousin of Banrith's from Cambodia. And when Banrith himself married Thangpin Somkhan in a traditional Cambodian ceremony, Walker's mother stood up for him as his surrogate mother, representing as well as she could the thirty-eight members of Banrith's family who had been executed or starved to death during the Pol Pot regime. Banrith and his wife have four children.

Stan Breen

Breen served as director of ARC until 1985 and remained on the board until his death in 1992.

Karen Johnson Elshazly

When she and Stan Breen sent the first ARC volunteers to Thailand in October

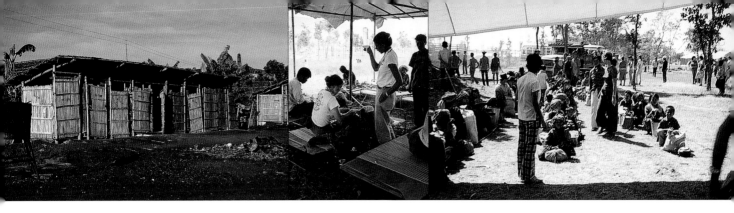

1979, "our goal was to put ourselves out of a job," Elshazly says. "We planned to work with refugees only until the Thai-Cambodian camps were empty." Twenty-eight years later, she's still there. The former director of operations who once shared a single office with Breen is now one of sixty-six staffers who direct the activities of 1,840 workers around the world. Elshazly works on planning issues, quality assurance, and security, and serves as ARC's corporate memory.

An evaluation of ARC in 1984 gave the organization its new direction and Elshazly a lifetime career. Consultants pointed out how extraordinarily effective ARC's health-care workers had been in the field, thanks to its revolutionary philosophy of education and prevention initiated by Dr. Steve Miles. Since the world tide of refugees had not diminished but increased, the consultants advised that ARC should not shut down but expand to work in other crisis areas throughout the world. "It was a turning point for the organization," remembers Elshazly, who is married and has one child.

Monorom Sok Hang
Monorom worked as an interpreter at the International Clinic for six years. He also enrolled at Lakewood Community College (now Century College) to further his education. "I had to take biology and chemistry," he says. "Pat Walker helped me write my essays in English, helped me with my

courses." He graduated from Century College as a registered nurse in 1996. After a stint at Regions Hospital, he has worked as a home-care nurse, specializing in the care of immigrants. Though he takes care of patients from all over the world, he has developed a specialty in Hmong health care. He and his wife, Naroeun, have two children. His sister, Rattana, is also married. His brother Mony married, has two children, and is now divorced.

Dr. Neal Holtan
For more than twenty years, Holtan practiced internal and preventive medicine in St. Paul, where in 1980 he founded what has since become the Center for International Health at Regions Hospital. He is the owner of Preventive Medicine Consulting and director of health-care practice for Partnership Continuum, a consulting firm that provides medical direction to the Minnesota Institute of Public Health. His particular interest is in environmental and social policy to prevent alcohol use among young people aged twelve to seventeen years. Holtan also serves part-time as medical director and tuberculosis physician at the St. Paul–Ramsey County Department of Public Health. He has been a physician with Minneapolis's Center for Victims of Torture from its inception in 1985. He is working on his doctorate in the history of medicine and public health, thanks to a 1998 Bush Medical Fellowship. He lives with his partner in Minneapolis.

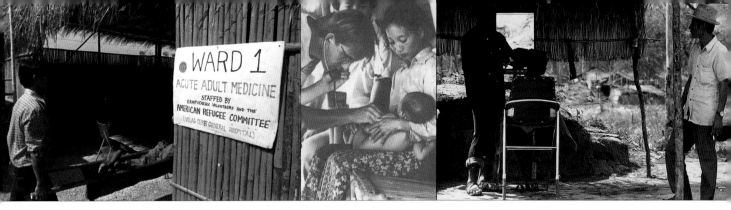

Barbara Huwe

As a result of her experience as an ARC 15 volunteer in Southeast Asia, Huwe became a Ramsey County public-health nurse as part of an international team. She now works full-time bringing services to the homes of people with disabilities, providing case management and making sure they live in a safe environment. She continues to be involved in peace and justice issues.

Xiong My Ly

Ly was one of the first two Hmong interpreters hired by Dr. Neal Holtan when he opened the International Clinic at St. Paul–Ramsey Medical Center. She did not retire from her position until 2006. Saying that she learned to speak English on the job, Xiong My Ly adds that she is most proud of her five children and the fact that her family never went on public assistance.

Dr. Steve Miles

Following his stint with the ARC 15 in Thailand, Miles came back to Minneapolis to finish his medical residency. In 1981 he returned to Thailand as ARC's medical director, a position he still holds, and tackled a problem that the World Health Organization had been unable to solve. Miles figured out a way to get patients to take TB treatment in an open air refugee camp that resulted in 98 percent patient compliance. The program has become the standard of care for refugees with TB, HIV, and other infectious diseases.

In Minnesota, Miles became an internist and geriatrician, as well as professor of medicine at the University of Minnesota Medical School and a faculty member of the university's Center for Bioethics and Council on Aging. He has served as chief medical officer for a Cambodian refugee camp, helped develop a medical school curriculum in Cuba, and focused on AIDS prevention in the Sudan. He ran, unsuccessfully, as a DFL Party candidate for the U.S. Senate in 2000. For his work in bioethics, public health, and human rights he received the 2000 Distinguished Service Award from the American Society of Bioethics and Humanities. Miles is the author of the universally acclaimed "Do Not Resuscitate" order.

In 2004 *Minnesota Monthly* magazine named Miles its "Man of the Year" after he single-handedly broke the story about the participation of military health-care workers in the torture of detainees at Guantanamo Bay and at Abu Ghraib prison. His book, *Oath Betrayed: Torture, Medical Complicity, and the War on Terror,* was published in 2006. He is married and has two daughters.

May Mua

Mua continues to work at the Center for International Health. Her son David, whose burns led Mua to become a nurse practitioner, is now entering college, and she has

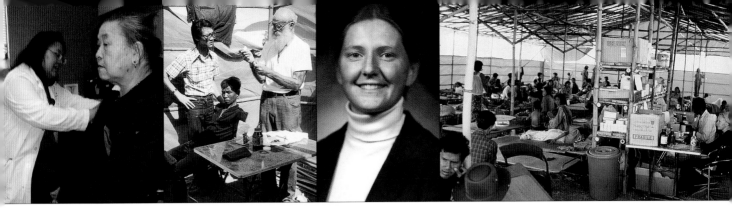

two teen-aged daughters. Mua herself is completing the demanding course on tropical medicine and hygiene at the University of Minnesota and will be certified in clinical tropical medicine and traveler's health, refugee, and immigrant health after she completes her two-month overseas residency and sits for the examination. She hopes to do her overseas work in Laos.

Diem Ngoc Nguyen

In 2005, the day after Nguyen retired from his eleven-year job as an interpreter at Regions Hospital, he and his wife, Thu, flew to Paris for his longed-for visit to France. His heart melted when the customs officer at Charles de Gaulle airport, after a brief glance at Nguyen's passport, smiled at him and said, "Welcome to France." Among the friends there to greet him were two diplomats and a physician who had been imprisoned with him, as well as former classmates from the Catholic school he had attended in Hanoi—men he had not seen since 1955.

The Vietnamese Association of Former Diplomats in Paris organized a party in Nguyen's honor. One of the guests was the foreign minister he had last seen thirty years before in the Riyadh airport. Nguyen had always been perplexed by the foreign minister's sudden departure from Saudi Arabia for Washington, D.C., while Nguyen returned to Vietnam and certain imprisonment. When Nguyen finished his remarks to the group, the foreign minister stood and for the first time spoke in public about the events that had occurred in Saudi Arabia and Washington in the days before South Vietnam's collapse. He told the group that he had been recalled to Washington at the last minute to assist the envoys already there in their final appeal for help to the U.S. Congress. When he finished speaking, he and Nguyen embraced. Nguyen calls it the happiest moment of his trip.

Nguyen has completed his annotated English-Vietnamese medical dictionary, a work of 1,005 pages, and is now compiling a second dictionary that lists medical terms in Vietnamese, gives the English expression, and then the French equivalent, along with an explanation of the illness or procedure. Nguyen devotes four to five hours a day to this project. His two children live in St. Paul. He and his wife have four grandchildren.

Monica Overkamp

When Overkamp returned from the Thai refugee camps, the nurse practitioner took a position providing primary care at the University of Minnesota Hospitals. In 1992 Pat Walker offered Overkamp a position at the International Clinic, soon to become the Center for International Health. She divided her time between the center and the U of M for several years, eventually taking a part-time position at the Health Partners Travel Clinic while also serving on the university's Department of Medicine faculty. Overkamp says that she still practices what she

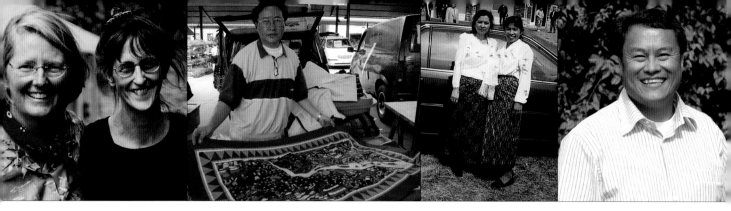

learned in the camps and at the Center for International Health with the large foreign-born population she sees in her current work. Overkamp is married and has three children, including a Korean adoptee.

Dr. Mikhail Perelman

Perelman continues to see patients at the Center for International Health. His daughter has become a registered nurse and, in June 2006, a mother. Perelman says he has already convinced his granddaughter to become a doctor. He has not changed his nationality on his passport, saying, "I have an American passport, but inside I am Russian." He has a satellite dish on his house that enables him to receive two channels of Russian TV and he follows Russian news daily. A large poster over his desk bears the likenesses of dozens of Russian heroes—politicians, poets, writers, and musicians.

Glenda Potter

Potter worked with the Legal Aid Society of Minneapolis for fourteen years before moving to the United Cambodian Association of Minnesota, where she writes grants and works on immigration and family reunification projects. She helped Channy and Veera Som compile the documents that allowed their remaining sisters and families—eleven individuals in all—to immigrate to the United States.

Channy and Veera Som

After they immigrated to Minnesota in 1990,

Channy says, the sisters felt compelled to help their family—their father, three sisters, and two brothers—who were still back in Cambodia. One brother immigrated to the United States soon after Channy and Veera arrived. A second brother and a sister died in Cambodia; Veera adopted their children, two boys and two girls, bringing them to the United States in the early 2000s, just before the program through which they were allowed to enter ended. Both sisters are married, Channy to a man she met in the Thai refugee camp who also became a medic trained by the American Refugee Committee. The couple has one daughter.

Mao Heu Thao

After graduating with a nursing degree in 1986, Thao joined the St. Paul–Ramsey County Department of Public Health, where she is now the Hmong health coordinator. Among the programs she initiated is the Hmong Health Care Professionals Coalition, a group of physicians, nurses, and other health-care professionals who address health concerns of the Hmong community. The coalition sponsors the Hmong Health Fair at the annual Minnesota Hmong Sports Festival, providing health education and screening. Thanks to a Bush Foundation Leadership fellowship, Thao also earned a degree in health education and program administration at Metropolitan State University in 1990. She is the former host of "Kez Koom Saib," a Twin Cities public television program that provides health-care information to the Hmong

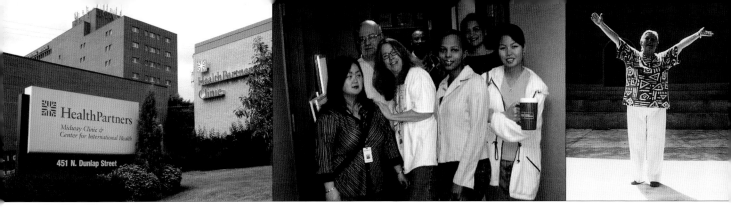

community. She now hosts "ECHO (Emergency Community Health Outreach)," which covers heatlh topics and emergency preparedness for her Hmong community. Her two children are graduates of American universities.

Bridget Votel

Votel continued as nurse manager of the Center for International Health until 2004, when she took a similar position with the United Family Practice Health Center, a federally qualified clinic in St. Paul. "I wanted to take what I had learned at the Center for International Health and use it elsewhere, expand it into the general practice," she explains. "I wanted to see it become part of the mainstream." Ideas first put into practice at the Center for International Health, such as staffing the clinic with providers from the same community that the organization serves and hiring professional medical interpreters, have become standard procedure at United Family Practice. Votel is also developing a cultural curriculum, based on the lessons she learned at the Center for International Health.

Frederick Walker

Walker's flying career spanned 24,850 hours and thirty years in Asia. He flew with the 14th Air Force over the Himalayas (the "Hump") in World War II with General Claire Chenault and Civil Air Transport in the Battle of Dien Bien Phu. He became chief pilot for Air America in Southeast Asia, flying in Laos, Cambodia, Thailand, and Vietnam until Apriil 1975. After flying in Egypt and the Bahamas, he retired

and lived in Maine and Florida until his death in 1999. His family donated his papers and aviation memorabilia to the Aviation History Museum at the University of Texas in Dallas.

Phyllis Walker (picured above right, arms outstretched)

Walker raised her five children in Taiwan and Thailand, often alone with other wives, all unsure of the safety of their pilot husbands. She learned to speak some Mandarin and Thai and was a gracious hostess, loving mother, and loyal friend. After her divorce and return to the United States, she worked as an employment counselor. She always opened her home and heart to her children's refugee friends and world travelers. She died in 1997 following a courageous sixteen-year battle against breast cancer.

Susan Walker

Walker stayed on in Thailand and for fifteen years served as the Southwest Asia director of Handicap International, a French NGO that organized workshops to make prostheses for land-mine victims. From Thailand she moved to Geneva, Switzerland, where Handicap International and five other nongovernmental organizations formed the consortium known as the International Campaign to Ban Landmines. Together with the consortium and its coordinator, Jody Williams, Walker was a co-laureate of the Nobel Peace Prize in 1997 for their efforts to ban land mines worldwide. Walker continues to live in Geneva as a humanitarian affairs and disarmament consultant with a focus on banning land-mine proliferation.

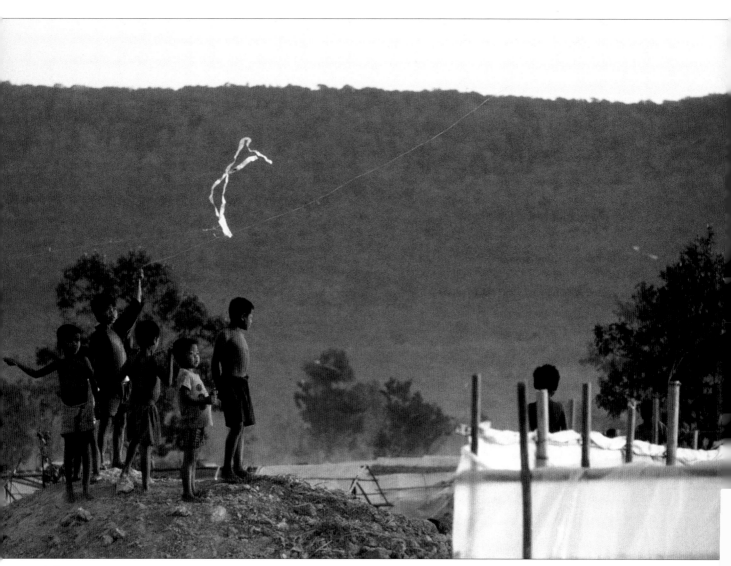

Children at the Khao I Dang camp fly handmade kites on a small hill by the camp latrines.

illustration credits

FOZIA ABRAR, M.D.,
Woodbury, Minnesota
p. 141, Dr. Fozia Abrar.

AVIVA BREEN,
Minneapolis, Minnesota
p. 30, Aviva and Stanley Breen with John Denver and adopted son.

CORBIS, www.corbis.com
p. 6–7, Somalia, Peter Turnley/COR-BIS; p. 112, French POWs, Bettmann/CORBIS; p. 114, Battle of Dien Bien Phu, CORBIS; p. 117, General Vang Pao, Bettmann/CORBIS; p. 139, Somalia, Peter Turnley/CORBIS; p. 140, Mogadishu, Patrick Robert/Sygma/CORBIS; p. 155 (bottom), Wat Tham Krabok, Darren Hauck/CORBIS.

DR. KATHLEEN CULHANE-PERA,
St. Paul, Minnesota
p. 24, altar.

KAREN JOHNSON ELSHAZLY,
Minneapolis, Minnesota
p. 35 (top), Karen Johnson Elshazly.

GETTY IMAGES,
www.gettyimages.com
p. 52 (bottom), Haing Ngor, Rob Boren/AFP/Getty Images; p. 96, Khmer Rouge, Claude Juvenal/AFP/Getty Images; p. 98, Cambodians fleeing Phnom Penh, AFP/AFP/Getty Images; p. 119 (top), Saigon's fall, Francoise De Mulder/Roger Viollet/Getty Images; p. 119 (bottom), North Vietnamese tanks, AFP/Getty Images; p. 155 (top), Mayor Randy Kelly, Pornchai Kittiwongsakul/AFP/Getty Images.

MONOROM SOK HANG,
Minneapolis, Minnesota
p. 102, Hang family; p. 103 (top), Monorom Hang, p. 103 (bottom), wedding.

DOUG HULCHER,
New York, New York
p. 70, Ban Vanai refugee camp.

MARK JENSEN,
Minneapolis, Minnesota
p. 104, farmers' market.

CHUCK JOHNSTON,
Afton, Minnesota
p. 12 and 34, story quilt; p. 190 (far right), Lee Pao Xiong.

JOANNE LANE, VISITED PLANET,
www.visitedplanet.com
p. 4, view toward Ho Chi Minh trail.

CAROLYN MCKAY,
Minneapolis, Minnesota
p. 62, pediatrician Carolyn McKay.

MINNESOTA HISTORICAL SOCIETY,
St. Paul, Minnesota
p. 60, Yong Vang Yang family, 1978 and 1979; p. 67 (top), graduating class, 1981; p. 67 (bottom), women sewing, 1983; p. 90, volleyball; p. 104, mother and son, Mark E. Jensen, 1998; p. 128, wedding reception.

ROBERT MULHAUSEN, M.D.,
Minneapolis, Minnesota
p. 26, St. Paul–Ramsey Medical Center; p. 65, Bob Mulhausen.

CHRIS NEWBERRY,
New York, New York
p. 16, clinic.

DIEM NGOC NGUYEN,
Roseville, Minnesota
p. 123, Diem Nguyen; p. 125–26, Nguyen family.

MONICA OVERKAMP,
Lino Lakes, Minnesota
p. 188 (second from left), Jeff Nelson.

MIKHAIL PERELMAN, M.D.,
Roseville, Minnesota
p. 129, Mikhail Perelman.

USN - DoD IMAGE
Front cover: Ghanaian girl.

BRIDGET VOTEL,
Minneapolis, Minnesota
p. 136 (top), Bridget Votel.

PATRICIA WALKER, M.D.,
Afton, Minnesota
p. 2, baby in bucket; p. 8, Pat Walker and Yong Yuth Banrith; p. 9, boat dock; p. 10, Ban Nong Samet camp; p. 11, Pat Walker and patient; p. 14, Laos; p. 20, Kathleen Culhane-Pera; p. 28, Pat and Susan Walker; p. 31, Neal Ball; p. 35 (bottom), Henry Kamm; p. 37, Susan and Pat Walker; p. 39, Fred Walker; p. 41–42, Ban Nong Samet camp; p. 44, Daniel Susott (top), refugees (bottom); p. 45, refugee family (top), man with rocket (bottom); p. 46, Cambodian brothers (top), patient

(bottom); p. 47–48, patient refugees; p. 49, Barb Huwe and patients; p. 50, Steve Miles; p. 51, Larry Kaplan and Pat Walker (top), Barb Huwe and staff (bottom); p. 52 (top), Haing Ngor; p. 53, Yong Yuth Banrith; p. 54, staff; p. 55 (top and bottom), refugees; p. 56, handmade toys; p. 57, girls at play (top), Steve Miles and Larry Kaplan (bottom); p. 58, Pat Walker; p. 61, Neal Holtan; p. 63, worms; p. 68, Mao Heu Thao; p. 70, Sao Kaeo camp; p. 72, Mao Heu Thao; p. 73, Xiong My Ly; p. 76, James Jaranson; p. 78, Cambodian monks; p. 80, Walker sisters; p. 81 (top and bottom), amputees; p. 82, graduating medics; p. 83, refugee medics (top), Pat Walker, Monica Overkamp, Monorom Sok Hang, Yan Yunn (bottom); p. 87, hut; p. 89, boat dock; p. 93, worm; p. 107, Jim Dixon, Elizabeth Walker Anderson, Xiong My Ly, Becky Enos; p. 108, Fartun Wardere (top), Channy Som (center), Sidney Van Dyke (bottom); p. 109, Mohamud Aden (top), Salvador Patino-Guzman (center), Kathy Jenkins (bottom); p. 110, Shelly Daohevang (top), Danglan Nguyen (center), Malinda Christopher (bottom); p. 111, Mardiya Jaffer (top), Soua Her (center), Georgi Kroupin (bottom); p. 113, Diem Ngoc Nguyen; p. 127, Diem Ngoc Nguyen; p. 136 (bottom), Basil Ivanov; p. 147, Karen Ta; p. 148, Bruce Field; p. 149, May Mua; p. 151, Angela Kuria; p. 154, staff; p. 156, Channy and Veera Som; p. 162, Ban Nong Samet; p. 164–65, Monica Overkamp and graduating medics; p. 167, French Doctors Without Borders hospital; p. 168 (top and bottom), Veera and Channy Som; p. 171, Glenda Potter with Veera and Channy Som; p. 172, Pat Walker; p. 174, Mikhail Perelman and patient; p. 184, coining; p. 185–91, Khao I Dang images; p. 192, Khao I Dang ; p. 196, grandmother and granddaughter; back cover.

WIKIPEDIA
p. 19, Mekong River.

BILOINE YOUNG,
St. Paul, Minnesota
p. 27, May Tho; p. 181, Pat Walker; p. 183, clinic images; p. 190 (second from left), farmers' market.

DAVID ZIEGENHAGEN,
Cloverdale, California
p. 40, David Ziegenhagen.

index

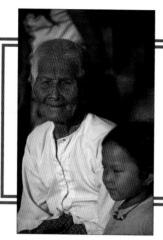

this book was designed
with care by

Mary Susan Oleson
NASHVILLE, TN